Pediatric
Palliative Care

Pediatric Palliative Care

Edited by

Lindsay B. Ragsdale and Elissa G. Miller

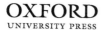

OXFORD
UNIVERSITY PRESS

OXFORD
UNIVERSITY PRESS

Oxford University Press is a department of the University of Oxford. It furthers
the University's objective of excellence in research, scholarship, and education
by publishing worldwide. Oxford is a registered trade mark of Oxford University
Press in the UK and certain other countries.

Published in the United States of America by Oxford University Press
198 Madison Avenue, New York, NY 10016, United States of America.

Library of Congress Cataloging-in-Publication Data
Names: Ragsdale, Lindsay B., editor. | Miller, Elissa G., editor.
Title: Pediatric palliative care / [edited by] Lindsay B. Ragsdale, Elissa G. Miller.
Other titles: Pediatric palliative care (Ragsdale)
Description: New York : Oxford University Press, [2020] |
Includes bibliographical references and index.
Identifiers: LCCN 2019035605 (print) | LCCN 2019035606 (ebook) |
ISBN 9780190051853 (pbk) | ISBN 9780190051877 (epub) |
ISBN 9780190051860 (updf) | ISBN 9780190051884 (online)
Subjects: MESH: Patient Care Planning | Pain | Palliative medicine |
Congenital | Developmental disabilities | Decision Making | Premature
Classification: LCC RJ249 (print) | LCC RJ249 (ebook) |
NLM WS 220 | DDC 618.92/0029—dc23
LC record available at https://lccn.loc.gov/2019035605
LC ebook record available at https://lccn.loc.gov/2019035606

9 8 7 6 5 4 3 2 1

Paperback printed by Marquis, Canada

Contents

Contributors

Toluwalase Ajayi, MD
Pediatric Palliative Care
Rady Children's Hospital
Scripps Research Translational
   Institute
San Diego, CA

Ricki Carroll, MD, MBE
Division of Orthogenetics
Nemours/Alfred I. duPont Hospital
   for Children
Wilmington, DE
Sidney Kimmel Medical College at
   Thomas Jefferson University
Philadelphia, PA

Mindy Dickerman, MD
Division of Critical Care Medicine
Division of Palliative Medicine
Nemours/Alfred I. duPont Hospital
   for Children
Wilmington, DE
Sidney Kimmel Medical College at
   Thomas Jefferson University
Philadephia, PA
Nemours/Alfred I. duPont Hospital
   for Children

Kelstan Ellis, DO, MS-CR, MBe
Section of Palliative Care
Children's Mercy
Kansas City, MO

David Flemig, MD
Adult and Pediatric Palliative Care
Children's Hospital of Colorado
University of Colorado Hospital
Aurora, CO

Jami Gross-Toalson, PhD
Department of Pediatrics
Department of Developmental and
   Behavioral Health
Children's Mercy
Kansas City, MO

Amelia Hayes, CCLS, MPH
Division of Palliative Medicine
Nemours/Alfred I. duPont Hospital
   for Children
Wilmington, DE

Natalie Jacobowski, MD
Child Psychiatry and
   Behavioral Health
Hospice and Palliative Medicine
Nationwide Children's Hospital
The Ohio State University College
   of Medicine
Columbus, OH

Emma Jones, MD
Pediatric Advanced Care Team
Dana Farber Cancer Institute
Boston Children's Hospital
Boston, MA

Carly Levy, MD
Division of Palliative Medicine
Nemours/Alfred I. duPont Hospital
  for Children
Wilmington, DE
Sidney Kimmel Medical College at
  Thomas Jefferson University
Philadelphia, PA

Jennifer Linebarger, MD, MPH
Section of Palliative Care
Children's Mercy
Kansas City, MO

Meghan L. Marsac, PhD
Division of Palliative Care
Kentucky Children's Hospital
University of Kentucky
Lexington, KY

Colleen Marty, MD
Pediatric Palliative Care and
  Pediatric Comprehensive Care
University of Utah
Primary Children's Hospital
Salt Lake City, UT

Elissa G. Miller, MD
Division of Palliative Medicine
Nemours/ Alfred I. duPont
  Hospital for Children
Wilmington, DE
Sidney Kimmel Medical College at
  Thomas Jefferson University
Philadelphia, PA

Dominic Moore, MD
Pediatric Palliative Care
University of Utah
Primary Children's Hospital
Salt Lake City, UT

Alexis Morvant, MD, MA
Children's Hospital New Orleans
  and Louisiana State University
  Health Sciences Center
New Orleans, LA

Laura Rose Musheno, MD
Perelman School of Medicine at the
  University of Pennsylvania
Pediatric Advanced Care Team
  at The Children's Hospital of
  Philadelphia
Philadelphia, PA

Cory Ellen Nourie, MSS, MLSP
Division of Transition Care
Nemours/Alfred I. DuPont
  Hospital for Children
Wilmington, DE

**Juliana H. O'Brien,
MSN, FNP-BC**
Division of Palliative Medicine
Nemours/Alfred I. duPont Hospital
  for Children
Wilmington, DE

Keith Pasichow, MD
Palliative Care Medical Director
Palliative Medicine Associates
Philadelphia, PA

Lindsay B. Ragsdale, MD
Division of Pediatric Palliative Care
Kentucky Children's Hospital
University of Kentucky
Lexington, KY

Megan J. Thorvilson, MD, MDiv
Comprehensive Pediatric and
  Adolescent Support Services
Mayo Clinic
Rochester, MN

Daniel Waechter Webb, MDiv
Spiritual Care Coordinator
Heartland Hospice
Traverse City, Michigan

Billie Winegard, MD, MPH
Section of Palliative Medicine
Phoenix Children's Hospital
Hospice of the Valley
Phoenix, AZ

Goals of Care

1 Whose Decision Is This?

Elissa G. Miller

You are caring for a 17-year-old with severe asthma who suffered a cardiac arrest 2 weeks ago, at which time she had a severe anoxic brain injury. Since the arrest, she has remained comatose with decerebrate posturing and persistent seizures. The consulting neurologist informs her parents that she is unlikely to ever regain consciousness and recommends ventilator withdrawal. Her mother states that she will "continue to pray" and we are "not stopping the machines. *Not now, not ever.*" However, her grandmother states that she had a conversation with her granddaughter a few months ago, in which they discussed a story in the news about a young girl who was kept alive on machines following a cardiac arrest. During that conversation, her granddaughter stated that if she were "ever in a permanent coma," she would not want to be kept alive on machines "like that girl in the news." The team calls you, worried that they do not know whose wishes to follow.

What do you do now?

SURROGATE DECISION-MAKING

A surrogate decision-maker is someone who makes decisions on behalf of a patient who is not able to make decisions for oneself. Most pediatric patients are not able to make their own medical decisions; therefore, the patients' parent(s) or guardian(s) acts as a surrogate decision-maker(s). This occurs by default in the care of minors, who, by definition, are not legally competent decision-makers. Parents are asked to make medical decisions based on what they believe is in their child's best interest. The best interest standard involves "attempting to determine what a 'reasonable person' would decide in a similar situation by weighing 'the burdens and benefits of treatment to the patient . . . when no clear preferences can be determined'" (Macauley, 2018, pp. 67–68). This differs from surrogate decision-making in adult care, in which decision-makers are asked to use substituted judgment. Substituted judgment asks the surrogate decision-maker to attempt to determine, as best as possible, what decision that person would make for themselves and is applied in the case of adults who once were able to make their own medical decisions but now cannot. But what about teenagers who are not yet their own legal decision-makers but who may have or have had the ability to state their own values and wishes?

As teenagers approach their 18th birthday, they are given an increasing voice in their health care, especially with regard to the use or refusal of permanent, life-prolonging technology and end-of-life care. In our case, the patient is still a minor, so her parents are her default surrogate decision-makers. Yet her grandmother reports information directly relevant to the decision at hand and may be able to make an informed, substituted judgment on her granddaughter's behalf. This is causing distress among the medical team members, who are worried about how to honor this patient's wishes when her family members disagree about what to do for her.

NAVIGATING DECISIONAL CONFLICT

In any case with decisional conflict, whether the conflict is between two surrogate decision-makers (i.e., parents) or between a surrogate decision-maker and another family member, as in our case, the ideal next step would be for the palliative care team or primary care team to have a family meeting to discuss the situation with all members of the family. The goal is to help all family members reach a consensus decision, weighing carefully the best interests of the patient, the patient's previously stated wishes when possible (substituted judgment), the family's goals of care for their loved one, and the medical team's recommendation. Often, in these situations, families are able to come to a unified decision—which in our case would mean either uniting behind her parents or her parents learning more about their daughter's wishes and honoring them despite her young age. It must be remembered that in the absence of family consensus, parents are still the surrogate decision-makers by law.

In our case, many would believe that her grandmother, who had the direct conversation with her granddaughter, would be the most appropriate surrogate decision-maker. However, this would not be allowed for a minor child without court intervention. The hospital could choose to pursue court intervention if it was believed that the parents were not acting in their daughter's best interests. Or her grandmother could petition the court for medical decision-making authority, arguing that if her granddaughter could communicate with us, she would tell us that she would not want to be kept alive on machines. If her family remains conflicted, or if one parent disagrees with the other despite active palliative care team engagement, an ethics consult can be helpful. This gives all parties, including members of the care team, a forum to discuss their concerns with a third party. Court intervention is a rare but sometimes necessary step if parents remain unable to agree on a treatment plan despite ethics and palliative care team involvement.

EMANCIPATED MINORS

In a few situations, minors may be emancipated—that is, freed from control by their parents or guardians—and allowed to make their own medical decisions. Partial emancipation occurs in many states surrounding sexual and reproductive health care. In addition, teenagers may petition the court to be emancipated; however, this is rare and frequently makes headlines when teenage patients choose to forgo medical treatment against the advice of their medical team. In the case of our patient, she is no longer able to speak for herself and so is unable to make her own medical decisions.

Where does this leave us? Although many believe a life on a ventilator is not the quality of life we would want for ourselves, this patient's mother is her surrogate decision-maker and is free to choose that for her daughter. It is not the recommended option; however, it is "not unreasonable" to continue life-prolonging medical therapies in the case of severe anoxic brain injury, and many families choose to do so. It would also not be unreasonable to discontinue the patient's ventilator and offer comfort care, given her devastating injury. A middle ground may be a time trial—a family may choose tracheostomy and mechanical ventilation for a period of time to determine their loved one's quality of life during the coming months. If they find that their loved one is suffering, they may choose to discontinue ventilator support at some point in the future. Although these situations are never easy, the role of palliative care in facilitating decision-making is crucial because it can help maintain an environment of mutual respect, even when opinions differ and families are in conflict.

KEY POINTS TO REMEMBER

- A minor's parent(s) or legal guardian(s) is their surrogate decision-maker unless ordered by a court.
- Other family members with knowledge of a patient's thoughts and wishes for their health care should be heard and the information weighed by the care team and the surrogate decision-maker(s); however, this does not alter decision-making authority.
- Teenagers are granted an increasing role in their health care decisions as they approach their 18th birthday. However, with the exception of sexual health or health care governed by local laws and emancipated minors, their parents remain the legal decision-makers until the day of the 18th birthday.
- A family meeting or ethics consult may be helpful if decisional conflicts arise.

Further Reading

Diekema DS. Parental refusals of medical treatment: The harm principle as threshold for state intervention. *Theor Med Bioeth*. 2004;25(4):243–264.

Macauley B. *Ethics in Palliative Care: A Complete Guide*. New York, NY: Oxford University Press; 2018.

Rhodes R, Holzman IR. Is the best interest standard good for pediatrics? *Pediatrics*. 2014;134(Suppl 2):S121–S129.

2 Why Is Everyone Giving up on Our Son?

Lindsay B. Ragsdale

You were asked to talk with parents in the intensive care unit (ICU) who are asking for full, aggressive care for their 8-month-old son, who has a rapidly progressive demyelinating disease. The infant has been declining during the past month in the ICU, with global weakness and long apneas requiring constant ventilator support. He started developing jerking and irritability at 2 months of age and now has progressive respiratory insufficiency. This week he was diagnosed with Krabbe disease, a progressive leukodystrophy that is usually fatal by 2 years of age. On exam, he is intubated with little spontaneous movement or response to stimulation and no cough or gag response. The parents are tearful, and they are wondering why everyone has given up on their son. You ask them about their understanding of his new diagnosis, and they say that a physician talked to them about the enzymes in their son's body and gave them some written information. They are angry and demanding answers.

What do you do now?

UNDERSTANDING CLINICAL ILLNESS

Due to the complexity of medical illness and the variety of information available, many patients and families have expressed feeling overwhelmed and have struggled sorting through medical information in order to make medical decisions. Especially with the large amount of information available online and in social media, maintaining clear communication and a concise plan of care can be challenging. Palliative care teams can assist families with understanding medical information and assess how they best receive information and match how medical information is given.

Medical training teaches clinicians to ask questions pertaining to patients' disease and symptoms, but this training commonly fails to prepare clinicians to assess how patients would choose to receive medical information. Assessing health literacy and communication preferences can be crucial to avoid miscommunications as in the clinical example. A simple question about how your patient or family likes to be communicated with can be very insightful. One physician shared her experience with an infant in the neonatal ICU with complex health issues. The patient had just been transferred from another hospital, and this physician asked how the mother would like to have medical information communicated. The mother shared that for the past 2 months at the other hospital, staff had been talking and writing to her in Spanish, but she does not speak Spanish; rather, she speaks a Mayan dialect and that has no written language. The physician discovered that she did not understand that her child had trisomy 21 and complex heart disease, but this conversation allowed for open communication in the appropriate language.

Many patients appreciate multiple routes of communication: verbal, written, drawings, medication charts, and troubleshooting guides. A father of a teenager with Duchenne muscular dystrophy asked the son's surgery team to create a paper outlining all of his medical problems and medications to share with first responders and emergency room clinicians. Although this father knew his son's medical issues completely, under stressful circumstances, he had difficulty remembering all the details. The American Academy of Pediatrics and the American College of Emergency Physicians have jointly published an emergency information sheet for children with special health care needs that can help clarify medial conditions in emergency situations. This same difficulty can occur in an inpatient unit with a medical team on rounds. Parents have commented that they feel overwhelmed sometimes by the number of people on rounds and that they forget everything they were going to ask. The use of a wipe board, journal for questions, or plan of care card can help parents remember their questions and the medical team communicate the daily plan. Other strategies are outlined in Table 2.1.

Some parents have different communication needs, and attending to these needs can help alleviate conflicts. A couple may have differing preferences—for example, one parent may prefer all the details, graphs, and literature; the other may be overwhelmed with all the data and withdraw. The team may discover this difference while asking about the parents' desire for medical information. They can attempt to arrange rounds to discuss the plan and broader medical status first for both of the parents to hear, and then the information-seeking parent can stay on rounds to ask the team more detailed, data-driven questions.

Some parents try to protect their sick child from hearing information about their illness as a way of preventing more stress. However, children as young as age 2 or 3 years may have questions about their medical illness and may want the opportunity to ask providers about their illness or procedures. Ensuring that medical information is given in a developmentally appropriate way is crucial for avoiding potential stress or medical trauma. If available, medical providers can use resources such as a child life

TABLE 2.1 **Strategies to Facilitate Illness Understanding**

- Query how patients/family prefer to receive medical information.
- Assess current level of understanding of medical illness.
- Use plain language and avoid medical jargon.
- Use simple drawings or pictures to help explain.
- Show images of radiologic scans and show a normal scan for comparison.
- Discuss the meaning of the illness with regard to daily life.
- Ask about hopes and fears when considering course of illness.
- Use an emergency information sheet for children with complex health care.

specialist, pediatric social worker, or pediatric psychologist to help tailor the information given to a child. Palliative teams can join with parents to have discussions with their child about the child's illness and can facilitate communication between them.

After assessing how patients and families wish to receive information, it is important to determine their level of understanding of the information that has been given so far. You can ask a question such as "I know you have been given a lot of information. What is your understanding of your daughter's illness?" The answer to this question can help you determine where you need to start in your explanation of the illness.

Often, there are cultural and/or spiritual implications to illness that can play a role in understanding of medical information. Medical teams should assess for cultural and spiritual influences in a thoughtful manner and approach families' beliefs with respect. Identifying and addressing these influences can help improve communication. Using resources such as chaplains, patients' spiritual leaders, and social workers can help elucidate spiritual and psychosocial dimensions to care.

Returning to the case example of the angry parents of the 8-month-old with Krabbe disease, the best first approach is to try to diffuse the anger and allow time to talk with the parents. You can use comments such as "I can see you are angry and upset. Would you mind helping me to understand what all you have been through with your son's illness?" After this discussion, you realize they did not understand the conversation with the physician who talked with them about enzymes. In fact, you learn that the parents struggle with their reading skills and they do not know what enzymes are or what this means for their son. You explain enzymes in a way they understand with a picture and an analogy to something familiar to them. You talk about the meaning of the new diagnosis and how this will impact his survival. The parents are tearful and devastated by the news, but they are no longer angry and understand what their son is facing. They decide to focus on their son's quality of life, and they make a plan for limiting painful procedures and getting him home.

- Inquire about caregiver's preferred communication modalities including language, literacy, written versus verbal, articles versus pictures, and details versus big picture ideas.
- Assess understanding of current illness and implications to quality of life in an empathetic way.
- Explore culture, spiritual, and psychosocial implications to illness and treatments and how this might impact care.
- Create educational materials geared toward the needs of the patient and caregivers.

Further Reading

Agency for Healthcare Research and Quality. *AHRQ Health Literacy Universal Precautions Toolkit*. Retrieved from https://www.ahrq.gov/professionals/quality-patient-safety/quality-resources/tools/literacy-toolkit/index.html

Marsac ML, Kindler C, Weiss D, Ragsdale L. Let's talk about it: Supporting family communication during end-of-life care of pediatric patients. *J Palliat Med.* 2018;21(6):862–878.

Miller VA. Involving youth with a chronic illness in decision-making: Highlighting the role of providers. *Pediatrics.* 2018;142(Suppl 3):S142–S148.

Nunstedt H, Rudolfsson G, Alsén P, Pennbrant S. Strategies for healthcare professionals to facilitate patient illness understanding. *J Clin Nurs.* 2017;26(23–24):4696–4706.

3 Will My Baby Learn to Walk?

Elissa G. Miller

You are called by a physician in the neonatal intensive care unit to meet the family of a newborn who was recently diagnosed with severe hypoxic ischemic encephalopathy following placental abruption and emergency cesarean section. The infant is now 3 weeks old. She is breathing comfortably on room air, although she is not taking a bottle well due to poorly coordinated suck–swallow–breath (SSwB) reflex. She also had an aspiration event last week not related to attempted feeding, and the team believes that she is at risk for recurrent aspiration. Her parents are wondering "what her life will be like" and want to know her prognosis for long-term survival.

What do you do now?

PROGNOSTICATION

Prognostication in pediatric palliative care can be extremely difficult. This is due to a number of factors, including diversity of underlying diagnoses, variability in medical trajectories, and limited prospective research. Neurologic prognostication, especially in the neonatal period, is even more difficult due to neuroplasticity of the pediatric brain.

In our case, as in many cases like it, we have some information that can help guide us in sharing the neurologic and overall prognosis for this patient:

1. Respiratory status: Our patient is breathing comfortably on room air, although a recent aspiration event indicates difficulty protecting her airway. This is a common area we look at when determining a patient's prognosis following anoxic brain injury or other neurologic diagnosis.

2. Oral intake: Our patient is unable to take a bottle due to a poorly coordinated SSwB reflex. For some infants, such as those born prematurely, this poor reflex coordination is temporary and their SSwB reflex becomes more coordinated as their brains develop. For others, this poor reflex coordination may be permanent. When poor SSwB is expected to be permanent, as it is likely to be for our patient, a gastrostomy tube for feeding is commonly recommended. Requiring a gastrostomy tube is associated with increased severity of cerebral palsy and subsequent decreased life expectancy, although this child could live for decades depending on the care decisions her family makes for her.

3. Developmental milestones: Although our patient is too young to have gained any developmental milestones, we would expect that she would begin making eye contact and develop a social smile within the next few weeks. Discussing with her parents the expected developmental milestones and any failures to meet these milestones over time may be helpful for them to gauge what developmental progress they can expect her to make.

4. Neurologic status: Our patient has had no seizures despite her severe brain injury. Seizures are common following anoxic brain

injury and portend worse prognosis when they are difficult to control or intractable. In addition to seizures, patients develop static encephalopathy following severe brain injury. From this, there is a slow decline over many years of the organ systems controlled by the damaged nervous system. Worsening autonomic dysfunction, progressive enteric nervous system dysfunction, and neurogenic bowel and bladder may all occur as a child with central nervous system injury ages. The earlier this organ system dysfunction arises, the worse the child's long-term prognosis.

Overall, this infant is unlikely to meet developmental milestones, but neuroplasticity of the developing brain leaves room for uncertainty. It is therefore reasonable to tell this family the following:

- We expect their daughter to be medically fragile all her life.
- Their daughter will show us what she can and cannot do. For some infants, we find this out sooner (they never meet any developmental milestones), and others develop a few milestones before reaching a plateau. This is something we will watch over time to help us assess her long-term prognosis.
- Her family will likely have difficult decisions to make in her future (e.g., those regarding repeated intubations with illness and future tracheostomy/ventilator dependence). Palliative care teams can help families think through these decisions as they arise or as we see them likely to arise in the near future based on clinical condition as children grow older.
- Some families reach a point where they believe their child's quality of life is so poor that they do not want to use life-sustaining technology to prolong their child's suffering. If a family gets to this point or starts asking questions about this topic, palliative care can discuss options for maximizing quality of life while not prolonging suffering with medical technology.

But what if a family is not asking for prognostic information? What if you have to share news of a poor prognosis with a family who has not yet been told what their child is facing? Or what if they do not believe the prognostic information you are telling them?

When a patient's prognosis is poor, many health care providers worry about taking away hope by sharing information about poor prognosis. However, data show that honesty from providers, even when a child's prognosis is poor, helps parents maintain realistic hope even in the face of devastating illness. Therefore, we strive for compassionate honesty when delivering news about poor prognosis.

To best support families when delivering news about poor prognosis, we often ask the following questions to help improve communication:

- How do you like to receive medical information?
- Is there anyone you would like to have here with you when we discuss difficult medical information?

These questions help us deliver news in a manner families are best prepared to hear. Some families will tell you they like to know "all the possibilities so we can be prepared." Others say they "want to take things as they come. One day at a time." "Give it to me straight." or "please don't talk about bad news when I am here alone." These are all answers families may give that tell us how best to communicate with them.

When preparing to deliver information regarding a poor prognosis for the first time, keeping in mind a family's preferred communication as established previously, there are a few cognitive frameworks, or mind maps, that may be helpful. Well-established cognitive maps, such as Buckman's SPIKES model (Table 3.1), have demonstrated improvement in provider performance and self-efficacy in navigating difficult conversations with adult patients. In delivering difficult news to pediatric patients and their families, providers utilize the same communication skills, adapted based on the developmental age of the child and the child's family system. Feudtner outlined a common-sense approach to these conversations (Figure 3.1) designed for pediatric use, although this map has not been studied in the same manner as the SPIKES model. Whichever approach you choose, utilizing a cognitive map can make the process easier for those delivering and for those receiving the information.

Despite our best attempts, not all families are as open in requesting prognostic information as was the family in our case, and many families will not believe the prognosis the team is presenting. This disbelief may be because of personal or family experience with incorrect prognostication, because of

TABLE 3.1 SPIKES Model

S Setting	Make sure you have the right people, including family members and members of the care team. Find the right location—someplace private and quiet where you will not be interrupted. Set up the room, including tissues or water that you may want to have available.	"Is there anyone you would like to have with you when we meet?" "Who from the care team is important for you to have at the meeting?"
P Perception	Solicit family's understanding of illness, including seriousness of the condition. Listen to the patient's level of understanding.	"What have you heard from the other doctors about how your child is doing?"
I Invitation	Ask the patient or family if they want to know more details about the medical condition. Ask if the family is ready to hear any important test results you have to present.	"Is it okay if I share with you some difficult news?" "Is now a good time to talk about what the team is worried about?"
K Knowledge	Share medical facts using simple language. Give information in small chunks with teach back to ensure understanding. Pause as needed to allow the family time to process information.	"Unfortunately, her scan shows the cancer is getting worse." "When we did the CT scan, it showed us she had a bad bleed in her head and that is why she is not waking up."
E Explore emotions	Offer an empathetic response. Identify emotion expressed by the patients. Ask patients to explain what they are feeling.	"Is hearing this news surprising to you?" "I can see that you are tearful. Tell what you are thinking about."
S Summary and next steps	Close the meeting. Ask if the family needs any additional clarification. Offer a next steps plan.	"This is not what any of us were hoping for. For now, we're not going to make any changes, but I'd like to meet again tomorrow to talk more about the plan moving forward." "I've shared a lot of difficult information with you. Would you like some time to talk as a family and I can come back in a few hours to talk more?"

Source: Adapted from Baile WF, Buckman R, Lenzi R, Glober G, Beale EA, Kudelka AP. SPIKES—A six-step protocol for delivering bad news: Application to the patient with cancer. *The Oncologist*. 2000;5(4):302–311.

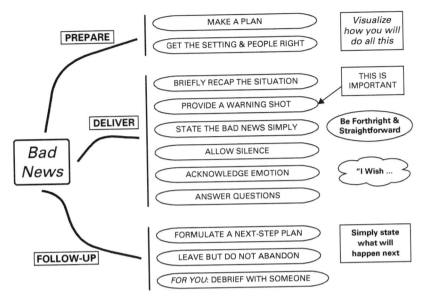

FIGURE 3.1 Feudtner's delivery of bad news.

Source: From Feudtner C. Collaborative communication in pediatric palliative care: A foundation for problem-solving and decision-making. *Pediatr Clin North Am.* 2007;54:583–607.

personal or religious beliefs, or because of distrust of the medical team or medical establishment. Offering a second opinion may be helpful for some families. Other families will need time to understand that the clinical team's prognosis was accurate (or inaccurate) before they can relinquish their mistrust. Leaving room for uncertainty when a prognosis is uncertain is as important as honesty when a prognosis is poor. This helps build trust with families and allows them to make fully informed decisions about their child's health care.

KEY POINTS TO REMEMBER

- Prognostication in pediatric palliative care remains difficult but there is information we can share with families to help them understand what we are looking at to determine prognosis.
- Neurologic prognostication is even more difficult due to the neuroplasticity of the developing brain.

- Discussing a range of future possibilities may be helpful to some families so they know what to expect. Others may prefer to "take things as they come."
- In situations where conflicts arise or difficult healthcare decisions must be made based on inadequate prognostic information, a second opinion may be helpful to aid decision making.
- Using a cognitive map helps with discussions about poor prognosis.

Further Reading

Baile WF, Buckman R, Lenzi R, Glober G, Beale EA, Kudelka AP. SPIKES—A six-step protocol for delivering bad news: Application to the patient with cancer. *The Oncologist*. 2000;5(4):302.

Feudtner C. Collaborative communication in pediatric palliative care: A foundation for problem-solving and decision-making. *Pediatr Clin North Am*. 2007;54:583–607.

Sisk BA, Kang TI, Mack JW. Sources of parental hope in pediatric oncology. *Pediatr Blood Cancer*. 2018;65(6):e26981.

4 We Are So Glad She Saw the Beach

Lindsay B. Ragsdale

A 3-year-old female with hydranencephaly is in the pediatric intensive care unit (ICU) with acute on chronic respiratory failure. You have been following this child for family support and chronic care since she was an infant. She had been doing well at home but has had three ICU admissions requiring prolonged intubation in the past 3 months. At her last admission, she was put on bilevel positive airway pressure (BiPAP) for home use and has needed to wear it around the clock due to hypoventilation and hypoxia. Her parents have been loving and thoughtful about each decision for their daughter, but now they are struggling with the decision between a tracheostomy with long-term home mechanical ventilation or comfort care with compassionate extubation. They meet with you to discuss this decision, especially because you have known her since she was an infant. They ask you directly, "If it were your child, what would you do?"

What do you do now?

GOAL-CONCORDANT CARE

Despite the increasing complexity in our health care system, we still strive to align the care we are able to provide with patient wishes and values. When the medical care that is given matches the goals of the patient or surrogate, this is called goal-concordant care. Goal-concordant care sounds simple; however, in practice it can be complicated and difficult to achieve because of the wide variation in patient and medical provider goals and values. Alignment of medical care and patient values necessitates clear communication about current medical status, prognosis, treatment options, and the implications for the patient's quality of life and functionality. Time and sensitivity should also be given to discussing and distilling patient and family values and wishes. Achieving goal-concordant care requires communication about topics that are difficult for patients, families, and providers and that may be avoided or deferred due to discomfort on both sides. Primary medical teams are encouraged to have conversations with patients and families to discuss their goals of care. Palliative teams can assist in these discussions utilizing their expertise in communication to advance the conversation about preferences, wishes, hopes, and fears.

Quality communication about goals of care can include discussions with patients and surrogates about past experiences in medicine, family values, communication preferences, emotions related to illness, burdens of treatments, spiritual and cultural beliefs, and wishes for the future depending on the course of disease. The conversations may need to happen over time and are best started prior to a crisis, if possible. Cultivating a trusting relationship is helpful in facilitating these conversations as these topics can involve a patient's experience over time. Involving a trusted medical provider, such as a primary care physician, in the conversation can provide context to the patient's history and perspectives. Allowing enough time for the patient and/or family to express their thoughts and feelings is crucial, especially with the tendency for pressured medical providers to interrupt patients or family members. Many patients and families are able to identify wishes and preferences with a facilitated discussion with questions aimed at helping them think through the decisions (Table 4.1).

Once patient and family goals and values have been discussed or identified, the next step is to put these goals and values in the context of

TABLE 4.1 Helpful Questions to Facilitate Goals of Care Discussions

How do you like to receive medical information? How much or how little?

What do you understand about your medical illness?

How much has your illness impacted you and your family?

What makes you most happy in your life?

What do you hope to happen in the future with your illness?

If your hope does not occur, what would you want to focus on?

What is your biggest fear/worry related to your illness?

What do you think is a good quality of life? Poor quality of life?

Who would you want to make decisions for you if you couldn't speak for yourself (18 years old or older legally in the United States)?

Are there things you want your doctors to explain more? Less?

How would you want to be cared for if you were in a coma? Vegetative state? Not able to breathe on your own? Heart was to stop? Dying?

the medical illness. If there are no decisions to make at the moment, then documenting the patient's and family's values can be helpful for future visits or if the clinical status changes. Ensuring that these values and goals are readily available to the patient, caregivers, primary care provider, and treating hospital can be helpful to align medical care with these values and goals. A variety of advanced directive documents are available online. In addition, many states have moved to portable advance directives (Medical Orders for Scope of Treatment [MOST], Physician Orders for Scope of Treatment [POST], and Physician Orders for Life-Sustaining Treatment [POLST]), which describe goals of care, code status, artificial nutrition/hydration, and antibiotics. These forms can go with patients when moving from facility to facility or facility to home and give guidance to emergency medical service providers about the patient's wishes for care in case of declining status. If medical decisions need to be made in a crisis, clinicians can help patients and families discuss goals of care and share professional recommendations based on clinical experience and available scientific evidence. Shared decision-making involves discussions of medical recommendations and patient/surrogate goals and values and how these two ideals can guide medical care.

Goal-concordant care can be achieved when both ideals align; however, there are times when conflict arises between medical providers and patients and families. There are times when patients might have two conflicting goals—for example, a patient with respiratory failure wants to live longer but also not use any respiratory machines. These personal goal conflicts need to be empathetically approached and explored further with attention to the natural course of illness and effects on quality of life. Other times, patients want to focus on comfort and be at home, whereas the medical providers believe there are more medical options to try but the options do not align with patient wishes. These conflicts are bound to arise in a system with patients and providers with individual preferences and experiences in life. Emphasis should be placed on patient and family wishes and helping them explore the benefits and burdens of medical decisions with the input of medical professionals.

The long-terms effects from having a sick child are still being researched in detail; however, emerging evidence indicates that parents whose child died under highly stressful events without the opportunity to say goodbye are at increased risk for complicated grief. The residual effects on the surviving surrogate could be deleterious if the care was misaligned with personal wishes or values. Medical providers intersect their patients at short intervals and do not always share the same life experiences, risk factors, or resilience traits as those of their patients and families. The decisions that parents make for their child can affect their bereavement long term and should be treated with respect.

Returning to the case example, the parents of the 3-year-old patient with hydranencephaly are grappling with decisions about tracheostomy and long-term home mechanical ventilation or compassionate extubation. As the physician that has known them the longest, you have established a trusting relationship over time. You sit down with them to explore how they are coping with her declining status and their goals of care. After some discussion, you ascertain that they are fully informed of the decision at hand and the benefits and burdens of each option. They want to know all the details of each option and explore what this means for their daughter's quality of life. You talk about watching her grow and what she has been able to accomplish, including a road trip to the beach, meeting her grandparents, and meeting her new baby brother. You also discuss what you have seen her go through with increasing difficulty breathing, breakdown of her skin with the BiPAP machine, more infections, worsening scoliosis, and less awake time. You share your worry that her body is declining and that in past discussions, they have stated that a tracheostomy and a ventilator do not provide the quality of life that they want for her. The tracheostomy and ventilator will assist her lungs but will not change her brain abnormality. They wanted to ensure they were always making decisions for their daughter and not to just delay their own grief. After exploring more about their goals, they want to focus on her comfort and allow her body to continue the shut-down process off the ventilator. They are interested in making her life meaningful by donating organs or tissues to other people in need. You listen to them as they recount the wonderful 3 years they have had together. You help facilitate her end-of-life care, change her code status to do not resuscitate, involve a child life specialist for memory-making activities, and coordinate with the organ procurement agency to ensure she receives care that aligns with the family's values.

Facilitating goals of care conversations can be challenging, emotional, and rewarding for patients and families and medical professionals. However, these conversations are a crucial component to ensuring goal-concordant care for patients. For patients with chronic illness, these conversations should occur at a non-crisis point with a provider who has the most trusting relationship with the family, such as a primary care physician or palliative team. If in a crisis, patient and family goals should be established and then a shared decision-making model combining goals of care and medical recommendations should be employed.

KEY POINTS TO REMEMBER

- Establish goals of care—hopes, wishes, fears, and preferences.
- Ensure understanding of medical illness.
- Give recommendations based on clinical experience and best evidence.
- Use shared decision-making.
- Align medical interventions and goals of care for goal-concordant care.

Further Reading

Jaaniste T, Coombs S, Donnelly TJ, Kelk N, Beston D. Risk and resilience factors related to parental bereavement following the death of a child with a life-limiting condition. *Children (Basel)*. 2017;4(11).

Kaye EC., Gushue CA, DeMarsh S, et al. Illness and end-of-life experiences of children with cancer who receive palliative care. *Pediatr Blood Cancer.* 2018;65(4):e26895.

Miyajima K, Fujisawa D, Yoshimura K, et al. Association between quality of end-of-life care and possible complicated grief among bereaved family members. *J Palliat Med.* 2014;17(9):1025–1031.

Sanders JJ, Curtis JR, Tulsky JA. Achieving goal-concordant care: A conceptual model and approach to measuring serious illness communication and its impact. *J Palliat Med.* 2018;21(Suppl 2):S17–S27.

5 Can You Go Change the Family's Mind?

Toluwalase Ajayi

You are asked to speak with the parents of a 2-week-old infant regarding the code status of their baby. Soon after birth, the infant began grunting and was taken to the neonatal intensive care unit (NICU), where she was found on head ultrasound to have multicystic leukoencephalomalacia. She aspirates all oral liquids, so a feeding tube was placed. Her course is complicated by anemia and a persistently high lactate, so mitochondrial disorder workup is pending. Even with the feeding tube, the infant still shows signs of aspiration with significant feed intolerance. Despite the fact that their daughter is critically ill, the parents keep asking when they can take her home. The team is worried that she has a high risk for a precipitous cardiopulmonary arrest. The NICU team has asked you to meet with the parents to discuss code status.

What do you do now?

A NOTE ON "CODE STATUS"

In medicine in general, the default code status is full code, and it has been for many decades. Currently, many different terms are used to indicate what should happen to a person who suffers a cardiopulmonary arrest, including do not resuscitate (DNR), do not attempt resuscitation (DNAR), and allow natural death (AND). Despite this, many pediatric providers report that they do not have or have not received sufficient training in resuscitation discussions.

CODE STATUS WITHIN GOALS OF CARE AND SHARED DECISION-MAKING

In pediatrics, code status is rarely, if ever, addressed outside of a serious illness or clinical decline. Thus, in the context of seriously ill children, these conversations should be held within an overall goals of care discussion in a shared decision-making model. Starting with a good assessment of the parents' understanding of their child's current medical condition, and what their hopes are for the medical interventions being discussed, is the foundation for having these conversations. Once those broader goals have been assessed and confirmed, it is important to remember that a "code"—cardiopulmonary resuscitation for someone who has died—is a medical intervention, for a specific situation, and nothing more. If, for some reason, code status has to be discussed outside of a broader goals of care conversation, then it must be approached as one would approach discussing any other medical intervention—that is, with an understanding of the emotionality associated with it. Emotion is a key component to why these conversations are so challenging.

WHY PARENTS' EMOTIONS MATTER IN THIS CONVERSATION

For parents, having a conversation about code status is an indication that there is something serious with their child's health. They understand that their child has a decreased chance of survival compared with other children. This is an incredibly challenging situation for any parent. This is a large part of why having these conversations is difficult for providers and parents alike. What is helpful, however, is understanding why parents might change their child's code status to DNR/AND. Parents make this choice primarily because they want to honor the quality of life of their child or because they understand what their child would want. Parents have noted that when they see signs of physical decline, such as fatigue and decreased interaction, they know that their child will not survive and they want to maintain a good quality of life for the time they have left. However, if parents do not perceive their child as suffering or nearing the end of life, they will be less inclined to make any changes because they want to give their child the best chance of survival. Understanding the parents' perception of their child and the emotions behind this perception is imperative to being able to have these discussions. It was best said by Maurer et al. (2010): "Clinicians who help parents to identify and be true to their values may alleviate parents' emotional distress and promote the maintenance of their personal integrity and dignity during extraordinarily difficult circumstances" (p. 3297).

WHY CLINICIAN EMOTIONS MATTER
IN THIS CONVERSATION

When considering less value-laden medical interventions—for example, an antibiotic for a viral infection—clinicians are able to clearly weigh the benefits and burdens to the patient and know that there is clear evidence to not use antibiotics for viral infections. Furthermore, clinicians can even consider the possibility that treating the patient with antibiotics is unlikely to benefit the patient in the long term but may have some short-term benefit to the patient and parent that is outside the guidelines and recommendations. This line of thinking becomes exponentially more difficult when considering the risks and benefits of cardiopulmonary resuscitation in pediatrics. This is due in part to the resiliency of children. Whereas the outcomes for pediatric patients experiencing an out-of-hospital cardiac arrest are extremely poor, for arrests that occur in the hospital setting, survival to discharge home is greater than 30%. That alone makes recommending a no code or AND for any pediatric patient extremely challenging. The emotional investment and compassion we as clinicians bring to these conversations also have a major impact on our ability to discuss the code status as a medical intervention. Death is permanent, and knowing that there is even the slightest chance that a child could survive to discharge may weigh on clinicians as they approach these conversations.

Contained with the emotion is also the fear that the clinician might say the wrong words or might even project that the family is not ready to address code status when in reality the clinician is the one not ready to discuss it. This might then lead the clinician to place the burden of making this decision solely on the surrogate decision-makers without providing any recommendations. It has been shown that not only do surrogate decision-makers want physician input in emotionally laden decisions but also shared decision-making is the best approach in addressing these conversations.

Other challenges include the options that exist within different pediatric institutions and confusion with regard to these options. One academic pediatric institution has up to five options on its code status order form: Partial Code, Full Code, Do-Not-Resuscitate/Do-Not-Intubate (DNR/DNI), Do-Not-Resuscitate/Do-Not Escalate (DNR/DNE), and Do-Not-Resuscitate/Comfort Care Only (DNR/C). Expansion of the DNR/AND option in this manner moves the code status conversation outside of the decisions surrounding the immediate arrest event and into a goals of care conversation in which preferences for overall care are evaluated. The term *code status* describes what type of intervention a health care team will conduct in the event of a cardiopulmonary arrest. A code status should not and does not address situations of pre-arrest cardiac or pulmonary distress (Figure 5.1).

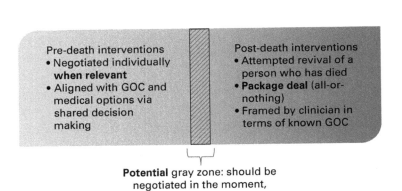

FIGURE 5.1 Parameters surrounding pre and post death interventions.

These considerations are addressed within the confines of a broader goals of care conversation and are difficult to place as an order. The expansion of the code status conversation to address goals of care also adds to the common misconception that the DNR/AND order means that a medical team will do nothing in the event of a patient emergency or that the patient will receive substandard care during the course of hospitalization. This is a concern and misconception that is held by both the caregiver and the medical provider, and it adds to the emotional burden that surrounds addressing code status.

All the previously discussed challenges arise from and are compounded by the limited amount of training that pediatricians receive on how to have these conversations. Given this, how does one approach a code status conversation?

APPROACH TO DISCUSSING CODE STATUS

Working with the case example, the following steps should be followed to address code status:

Step 1: Perception: This allows you to start from a good foundation of what the parents have processed from the information they have been given.

"[Parent's names], I know that you are eager to take your daughter home, and we want that as well. Can you please tell me what you understand about your daughter's overall health?"

- The parents at this point will either have a good general understanding or not, or even more complicating, you learn that the parents have two different perceptions about their child's current condition.

Step 2: Prognosis: Acknowledge the response you receive and provide a simple overall prognosis by stating the concern of the medical team. This is in general one of the most difficult steps because prognosis is so uncertain, and we as clinicians feel as though we must have all the information and be certain. This is not the case.

"You are correct, your daughter is stable right now, but she is still very sick, and I want to talk to you about what would happen if her heart were to stop beating or she was to stop breathing."

Or

"She does look really comfortable right now, she has made some
improvements, and we hope that these continue. We do worry
that despite all these improvements, she is still very sick, and
I want to talk to you about what would happen if her heart were
to stop beating or she was to stop breathing."

Or

"Her health is really complicated, and I can understand that you
must have heard a lot of confusing information. Overall, she is
currently stable, and we hope that she continues to improve, but
even with improvements she is still very sick, and I want to talk
to you about what would happen if her heart were to stop beating
or she was to stop breathing."

- These are sample phrases that allow you to acknowledge the
variety of responses you can receive from the parents, but they
keep you focused on the one topic you are discussing and the
prognosis related to that one topic.

Step 3: Describe cardiopulmonary resuscitation as a single, packaged
intervention: Use simple terms and state the risks and benefits as
they relate to the patient as concisely as possible.

"When a child's heart stops beating, or she stops breathing, we do
our best to start them back up again, hoping that we bring the
child back to life again. This involves pressing on the chest hard
enough that we can help the heart to start pumping again, using
medications to help the heart start pumping, and putting in a
breathing tube like your daughter has right now. It does cause
some harm to the child, but typically we feel that this harm is ok
if it can help that child live again."

Step 4: Physician recommendation: This is the part that will bring up a
variety of emotions for the clinician, and it is the most difficult. But
physicians need to be able to make a recommendation to the patient
based on their clinical expertise (Figure 5.2) and allow space for the
patient or the patient's surrogate to respond.

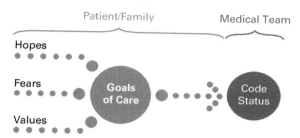

FIGURE 5.2 Addressing code status within a shared decision making model.

"Because of your daughter's illness, I worry that her body would not be strong enough to survive that trauma, and would recommend instead, that, if this ever happens, we do everything we can to ensure that she does not suffer, and she dies peacefully."

- It is important to address the patient's body, not the patient, that is not strong enough to survive. It is also important to note that there was no certainty in the previous recommendation, just a concern based on the clinical status of the child, shared by the medical team. There is no way to truly know for sure if, despite all her medical conditions, this patient will be among the 30+% of patients who survive an in-hospital arrest.

- After you give this recommendation, it is important to be silent and allow the family to respond. Either they accept your recommendation or, more likely, push back with more questions.

- It is usually during the questions that we as clinicians feel the pull to then offer more options and veer outside of the arrest situation. It is important to remember that the code status conversation is only in the case of a cardiopulmonary arrest. It is important to say to the family, again, that this is only if her heart were to stop or if she were to stop breathing. Until that point, a statement such as "We will continue to do everything we can to treat her health conditions" lets the family know that you are still actively caring for their daughter and that they are not being abandoned.

KEY POINTS TO REMEMBER

- Code status should be addressed within the overall goals of care for children with serious medical illness.
- Code status only addresses cardiopulmonary arrest events.
- Cardiopulmonary resuscitation should be described as a medical intervention.
- Patient/surrogate perception of the underlying condition and physician recommendation are key components to a successful approach.

Further Reading

Durall A, Zurakowski D, Wolfe J. Barriers to conducting advance care discussions for children with life-threatening conditions. *Pediatrics*. 2012;129(4):e975–e982.

Edmonds KP, Ajayi TA, Cain J, Yeung HN, Thornberry K. Establishing goals of care at any stage of illness: The PERSON mnemonic. *J Palliat Med*. 2014;17(10):1087.

Kim YS, Escobar GJ, Halpern SD, Greene JD, Kipnis P, Liu V. The natural history of changes in preferences for life-sustaining treatments and implications for inpatient mortality in younger and older hospitalized adults. *J Am Geriatr Soc*. 2016;64(5):981–989.

Maurer SH, Hinds PS, Spunt SL, Furman WL, Kane JR, Baker JN. Decision making by parents of children with incurable cancer who opt for enrollment on a phase I trial compared with choosing a do not resuscitate/terminal care option. *J Clin Oncol: Official J Am Soc Clin Oncol*. 2010;28(20):3292–3298. doi:10.1200/ JCO.2009.26.6502

Stevenson EK, Mehter HM, Walkey AJ, Wiener RS. Association between do not resuscitate/do not intubate status and resident physician decision-making: A national survey. *Ann Am Thorac Soc*. 2017;14(4):536–542.

Weise KL, Okun AL, Carter BS, Christian CW. Guidance on forgoing life-sustaining medical treatment. *Pediatrics*. 2017;140(3):e20171905.

Wolfe J, Klar N, Grier HE, et al. Understanding of prognosis among parents of children who died of cancer: Impact on treatment goals and integration of palliative care. *JAMA*. 2000;284(19):2469–2475.

6   In the Eye of the Beholder

Elissa G. Miller

You have a long-standing relationship with a child
who has severe neurologic impairment due to
mitochondrial (Leigh's) disease. At your last visit with
this patient and family, his parents believed that he
still has a good quality of life; he no longer talks,
but he enjoys listening to music and smiles when
his siblings are around him. They know that they do
not want him kept alive on a ventilator "if he is a
vegetable," but they continue to want aggressive, life-
sustaining treatments as long as he remains at his
cognitive baseline. He was admitted yesterday to the
intensive care unit (ICU) with respiratory failure due to
aspiration pneumonia. Although he is likely to survive
with aggressive intervention, the ICU team is not sure
that aggressive intervention is in the patient's best
interest. The ICU team is worried that this child has
"no quality of life" and calls asking you to talk to his
parents about discontinuing life-sustaining therapies.

What do you do now?

QUALITY OF LIFE

The World Health Organization (n.d.) defines *quality of life* (QOL) as "an individual's perception of their position in life in the context of the culture and value systems in which they live and in relation to their goals, expectations, standards and concerns." The American Centers for Disease Control defines *health-related QOL* as "an individual's or a group's perceived physical and mental health over time."

From these definitions, it is easy to see that QOL is a subjective measure. What one person defines as a good QOL, another person may define as a poor QOL. Our case is a common occurrence in modern health care: The health care team often assesses patients who require total care for all activities of daily living as having a poor QOL. Yet patients and families often assess the same clinical scenarios very differently.

In adult health care, most patients are able to tell you their QOL and if there have been changes over time with changes in their health status. Patients and their providers are then able to make clinical decisions in part based on QOL. However, in pediatrics, we are most often asking the child's parents to tell us about their child's QOL. And in the case of our patient, we are asking the parents to assess QOL for their nonverbal child who cannot participate in the conversation in any way. So how do we assess QOL?

ASSESSING QUALITY OF LIFE

There are many validated health-related QOL surveys that clinicians and researchers use to assess QOL, including the PedsQL. These surveys are useful screening tools in an ambulatory setting and can be helpful in prompting discussion. However, talking with a patient and the patient's family/surrogate decision-maker is the preferred method of assessing QOL in palliative care. We commonly ask the following questions to help us better understand a family's assessment of their loved one's QOL:

- What are their good days like?
- What are bad days like?
- How often are they having good days versus bad days, and has that changed over time?
- How is their quality of life?

- Have you noticed any changes in their quality of life?
- Do you think they are suffering?

Answers to these questions can help guide the conversation. For a pediatric patient whose surrogate decision-maker assesses a good QOL, care teams will often continue with life-prolonging therapies, even if the care team assesses the patient's QOL differently. However, if a patient or their caregiver assesses a poor QOL, we must now start to consider QOL in the context of patient prognosis. Is the poor QOL temporary, such as during cancer treatment for a patient with a high likelihood of cure? Is the poor QOL permanent, such as after suffering severe anoxic brain injury following a near-drowning event? Or is the poor QOL waxing and waning with disease exacerbations, such as in congestive heart failure, but with an expectation of continued downward decline as the disease progresses? Examining QOL in conjunction with patient prognosis can help providers and families set realistic expectations for the future. It also helps us assess if QOL may be utilized as a reason to alter our plan of care. That is, for a child with a good prognosis for long-term survival, such as a 5-year-old with newly diagnosed pre-B cell acute lymphoblastic leukemia, discontinuing medical therapies because of poor QOL is *not* an option because the poor QOL is expected to be transient with greater than a 90% chance of cure. However, for a child with incurable illness, such as end-stage congestive heart failure with no further surgical options, limiting aggressive interventions due to poor QOL is a reasonable therapeutic option.

USING QUALITY OF LIFE TO DETERMINE A CARE PLAN

For some families, QOL may help you determine a medication plan. For example, if a child undergoing cancer treatment has a poor QOL due to nausea, altering the patient's antiemetic regimen may improve their QOL significantly. Or for a child with significant neurologic impairment who has retching with gastric tube feedings, transition to jejunal tube feeds may improve their QOL. Both of these can be done without altering the overall disease trajectory.

In our case, the clinical team assessed poor QOL for the patient and wants to use this assessment to modify the care plan (i.e., discontinue life-sustaining technologies). However, you know the family has previously assessed their child to have a good QOL and one worth preserving using medical technology. So, in this clinical scenario, appropriate next steps would be to talk with the family. Ask them how things have been at home prior to this hospitalization. Has anything changed in their QOL assessment for their child? If nothing has changed, and their child still has a good QOL at home, this family may want to use all available life-prolonging technology to try to return their child to pre-hospital baseline. However, if the family has perceived declining QOL at home, they may want to discuss limiting medical interventions during this acute illness. Of course, it is important never to make assumptions and always to ask a family if their wishes for their child have changed.

KEY POINTS TO REMEMBER

- Quality of life is subjective.
- In palliative care, a discussion with the patient and/or family is the best way to assess quality of life.
- Prognosis must also be considered when using quality of life to help establish or change a plan of care.

Further Reading

Janse AJ, Gemke RJ, Uiterwaal CS, van der Tweel I, Kimpen JL, Sinnema G. Quality of life: Patients and doctors don't always agree: A meta-analysis. *J Clin Epidemiol.* 2004;57(7):653–661.

Janse AJ, Uiterwaal CS, Gemke RJ, Kimpen JL, Sinnema G. A difference in perception of quality of life in chronically ill children was found between parents and pediatricians. *J Clin Epidemiol.* 2005;58(5):495–502.

PedsQL. *The PedsQL measurement model for the Pediatric Quality of Life Inventory.* Retrieved May 30, 2019, from https://www.pedsql.org/index.html

World Health Organization. *Health statistics and information systems.* n.d. Retrieved May 30, 2019, from https://www.who.int/healthinfo/survey/whoqol-qualityoflife/en

7 You Can't Tell Him That!

Elissa G. Miller

You are called by a cardiologist to meet a 17-year-old male with Duchene muscular dystrophy and end-stage heart failure due to cardiomyopathy. The patient has previously declined ventricular assist device placement because he "does not want to be kept alive on machines." He is now experiencing dyspnea at rest with an ejection fraction of 7%. His cardiologist recommends hospice, and his parents are in agreement. However, his parents do not want you to tell their son that he is going home with hospice because they are worried he will "give up hope and die faster."

What do you do now?

TRUTH TELLING IN PEDIATRIC PALLIATIVE CARE

Truth telling, also known as prognostic disclosure, has not always been the norm in American health care. It was not until the 1960s and 1970s that physician opinion changed from largely preferring not to disclose diagnoses such as cancer to nearly universally disclosing diagnoses to patients in the United States. Truth telling for pediatric patients lagged further behind. Fear of confusing children or taking away hope led parents and providers to continue to prevent prognostic disclosure in pediatrics until the 1980s. Yet despite the pendulum swing for providers, from shielding patients from knowing to calling for more open and direct communication with children about prognosis, many parents remain resistant to the idea.

Parents often serve as gatekeepers of medical information flow to their children. This is appropriate for young children, such as those who are elementary school age or younger, because they are not making their own medical decisions and so do not need full prognostic disclosure at any time during their illness. However, as children become adolescents, the appropriateness of sharing medical information changes. And when discussing prognostic disclosure with dying children, providers sometimes join parents in their discomfort and gatekeeping. Yet children, especially adolescents, report wanting to know their prognosis even if the prognosis is poor. This aids in establishing realistic hopes and goals even as disease progresses. Most patients consider prognostic information to be extremely or very important. In one oncology study, more extensive prognostic disclosure with adolescents and young adults had higher odds of trust, peace of mind, and hope related to physician communication. Disclosure was also associated with lower distress related to knowing about prognosis.

However, children's understanding of illness and death evolves over time, and each child is unique in their development. Therefore, a child's developmental level is important to keep in mind when discussing prognostic disclosure. Adolescents should be given a choice whether to participate in the initial news-sharing conversation or to speak with the care team separately after the caregivers have received the news. The transition to full involvement in conversations may be very difficult for some teens, especially if they have been chronically ill throughout childhood and are used to their parents making medical decisions for them. It is often the role of the palliative care team to support and encourage prognostic disclosure with children of all ages at each child's developmentally appropriate level.

EXPLORING PARENT CONCERNS

When a parent asks you not to disclose medical information to their sick child, the best next step is to explore the parent's concerns:

- I'd like to talk more about this.
- Tell me what you're worried about?
- What do you think may happen if I tell him or her?

Sometimes the request is practical, such as "He has friends coming to visit and he has been really looking forward to that visit. I'd like to wait until after to tell him this news so he can enjoy the visit." Other times, it is based on knowledge of their child: "She said she prefers to hear that news from me [her parent]." These requests should be honored by clinicians. Other times, however, the request is rooted in fear—"What if he thinks I'm giving up on him?"—or family history—"The doctor told my mother she was dying and she just gave up and died a week later. I don't want that to happen to my daughter." Exploring family concerns about prognostic disclosure can open unexpected avenues of discussion. It is important for providers to listen to family's fears and validate concerns regarding how difficult these conversations can be. Providing families with the words to use when discussing prognosis with a dying child may be helpful. Also, families may want to hear provider experience with disclosing prognosis to children and teens. Letting families know that they do not need to say everything in one conversation is important; this can be an ongoing discussion with news delivered in manageable pieces as the child shows interest in knowing and talking more. In addition, we know from the literature that parents who have open conversations with their dying child do not regret it, even when the conversation is about death. So helping families navigate these important conversations is a valuable role of the palliative care team.

Yet sometimes parents continue to refuse to have an open, developmentally appropriate conversation with their dying child. What then? It is important for parents to know that the health care team will not lie to their child. If asked directly "Am I dying?" providers will reflect the question back at the child (e.g., "Why do you ask that?"), explore the child's concerns (e.g., "Is there something you're worried about?"), or deflect (e.g., "Is that something you've talked to your parents about?"), but providers will not lie. Most parents can accept that this is important in helping their child maintain trust in their provider. And most providers can honor parents' wishes about not offering prognostic information unless asked directly by the child, especially for young children. But what about a teenager, as in our case example?

ETHICS OF WITHHOLDING PROGNOSTIC DISCLOSURE

There are a few situations in which withholding prognostic disclosure raises ethical questions and concerns. Care of teenagers, as in our case, is one of those situations. Anyone aged 18 years or older needs to be asked directly by the provider if they want to hear more information about their illness. If a young adult, older than age 18 years, declines to hear more but is able to select a surrogate decision-maker (e.g., "Just tell my mom. She can make all my decisions for me. I don't want to know"), it is their autonomous right to decline to hear medical information and that request should be honored by the medical team, regardless of the age of the patient. What a young adult cannot do is decline to hear medical information and also decline to name a surrogate. Someone must make informed medical decisions for the patient, but it does not need to be the patient him- or herself. It would also not be ethical for parents to prevent providers from speaking with a competent 18-year-old unless or until the young adult has stated that they do not want to hear medical information. But what about a 17-year-old, as in our case? The patient in our case is still a minor, so his parents are making his medical decisions. But is it ethical, based on parental request, to withhold prognostic information from a patient who is nearly an adult? Despite being younger than the age of legal competence, our patient has already been involved in his medical decision-making in the past—he declined ventricular assist device because he "does not want to be kept alive on machines." So his parents and his providers have trusted his decisional capacity in other, difficult situations. Withholding his prognosis may prevent this patient from making plans to enjoy as best he can the time he has left, such as a final trip to the beach or a party with friends and family. Therefore, with-holding information may do harm. The benefits of prognostic disclosure, as discussed previously, include improved trust in providers and decreased anxiety. So is this a situation in which a provider would be justified in overriding parental wishes? It may be, but not without parents knowing of the provider's intentions:

> I understand your concerns, but he is old enough that he deserves to know. He has handled very difficult medical information in the past. I know we can support him through this. Would you like to be there when I talk with him?

Reassuring parents that you will not tell their minor child any more than the child wants to know is important: "I will let him lead the conversation. I will ask him how much he wants to hear and will honor his request if he does not want to talk about it."

HAVING THE CONVERSATION

Disclosing prognosis to an adolescent or young adult should start with a question: "How much do you know about what is going on with your disease and how much do you want to know?" Answers range from "I know I'm getting worse. My mom doesn't think I know. But I can feel it. Can you help me?" to "I dunno. Not much, I guess. Is my cancer back?" The next step is to tell the patient what he or she is asking for: "I think we can help you feel better, but the medicines are no longer helping your heart work better." Or "Yes, unfortunately, your cancer is back." Repeating the cycle (ask "Is there more you want to know?" and tell the patient what he or she is asking) is an easy way to have a patient-led conversation. The provider tells the patient only what he or she is asking to know.

For school-age children, a very serious question such as "Am I going to die?" may be best answered with a question: "That's an important question. Why are you asking me that?" The child's answer will help guide your next steps. An answer such as "Because my mom is crying a lot and she cried a lot when my grandma was dying" may lead to a more serious conversation. But a superficial response such as "Because all people die, right?" shows the child is still very concrete in his or her thinking.

When talking with our patient, he answered, "I know my heart is sicker. And my friend from muscular dystrophy camp died when his heart got worse. So I guess, maybe my time is coming." You explore more about his friend and learn that he visited his friend when he was home with hospice, dying. He understands that all patients with muscular dystrophy die young unless they choose to live on machines, which he reiterates that he does not want to do. Through this conversation, you are able to explore his hopes and his fears and set realistic goals for him to accomplish. He is tearful, but thanks you for being honest with him. He adds, "I hope my mom isn't mad at you for telling me." You let him know that you discussed this with his mom, and she "loves you and wants the best for you, even if that means hearing difficult news."

KEY POINTS TO REMEMBER

- Truth telling in pediatrics should occur in a developmentally appropriate way for each child.
- Parents appropriately serve as gatekeepers of medical information flow to school-age children and those who are younger. However, adolescents should be given a choice about how much they would like to hear from their provider.
- When a family is adamant about not disclosing prognosis to their child, providers should do their best to honor the request if it is ethically appropriate.
- Patients older than age 18 years may decline to hear prognostic information as long as they select a surrogate decision-maker who receives full medical information from providers.

Further Reading

Kreicbergs U, Valdimarsdóttir U, Onelöv E, Henter JI, Steineck G. Talking about death with children who have severe malignant disease. *N Engl J Med.* 2004;351:1175–1186.

Mack JW, Fasciano KM, Block SD. Communication about prognosis with adolescent and young adult patients with cancer: Information needs, prognostic awareness, and outcomes of disclosure. *J Clin Oncol.* 2018;36(18);1861–1867.

Sisk BA, Bluebon-Langner M, Wiener L, Mack J, Wolfe J. Prognostic disclosures to children: A historical perspective. *Pediatrics.* 2016;138(3):e20161278.

8 You Can't Stop the Machines!

Elissa G. Miller

You are caring for a child who is undergoing induction chemotherapy for newly diagnosed secondary acute myelocytic leukemia after having recently completed treatment for meduloblastoma. While neutropenic, he developed Stevens–Johnson syndrome, likely due to routine Bactrim prophylaxis. He developed acute respiratory distress syndrome requiring intubation and high-flow oscillatory ventilation. He has multiple chest tubes with persistent air leak, and after many weeks on the oscillator, he remains neutropenic and has shown no sign of improvement. He frequently becomes unstable, requiring medical resuscitation, and the team is in complete agreement that he will not survive his illness. The intensive care team recommends a do not resuscitate (DNR) order; however, his mother insists that you "do everything" and will not permit discussion of limitations of care.

What do you do now?

WHEN PARENTS WANT YOU TO "DO EVERYTHING"

The phrase "do everything" is one that gets uttered with unfortunate frequency when patients are critically or terminally ill. Sometimes it is said by well-meaning providers—"Would you like us to do everything?" Other times, as in our case, it is the family who insists that "everything" be done for their child. As and Chris Feudtner and Wynne Morrison (2012) outlined,

> We simply cannot do everything. There are so many—almost too many—possibilities. Medical care can go in many different directions, but not all at the same time. One cannot simultaneously cradle a grievously ill infant in one's arms and at the same time insert vascular cannulas for extracorporeal membrane oxygenation; nor can one hold a loved one's hand while they are dying at the same moment that the code team yells "clear" and attempts to defibrillate the patient's heart. One must choose. Whether acknowledged or not, choices are woven throughout the fabric of medical care. (p. 694)

So how can we help a family who is asking us to "do everything"?

As with much of our work in palliative care, the first step is to gather one's interdisciplinary team to meet with the family and understand their view of their child's illness. Do they fully understand their child's illness and prognosis? Or are there gaps in their understanding? Once a good understanding of the patient's illness has been established, the next step is establishing goals of care. A number of questions can be asked to help establish goals of care, including the following:

- "Given everything your child is up against, what are you hoping for?"

   Families will sometimes give initial answers that do not give the provider significant insight, such as "I'm hoping the doctors are wrong and my daughter survives." Asking further questions, either "What else are you hoping for?" or "If the doctors are not wrong, what are you hoping for?" may be helpful to draw families to a place where they can focus on the hope that exists even as a child's death becomes a certainty. Families often hope their child is comfortable, hope for more time, or hope they make or are making the right decisions. Helping families find what they are hoping for beyond the hope for their child's survival is often helpful in the beginning to establish goals of care.

· "What are you most afraid of?"

Families who are afraid their child is suffering, afraid of making the wrong decisions, or have any number of other fears regarding end of life are opening up a deeper discussion regarding goals for their child's care. How can the medical team help avoid the pain and suffering a family is worried about? How can the team help a parent feel confident in his or her decisions? However, not all families can have this discussion. Some families answer "I'm afraid my child will die" and cannot think beyond that fear. Other issues may come into play, as well, in establishing goals of care for a dying child. Family mistrust of the medical system, religious or spiritual beliefs, cultural differences, or a lack of trust in one or more providers may make families more resistant to discussing the reality of their child's situation. In these circumstances, it is important to rely on all members of the palliative care interdisciplinary team (IDT). Perhaps the chaplain can begin working with a family with strong religious beliefs to understand their theology and how that is affecting their decision-making. Perhaps the social worker can work with the family to better understand cultural differences. Working as an IDT helps us support the family's emotional and spiritual suffering as their child's life is nearing its end.

· "You said you want us to 'do everything.' What does 'do everything' mean to you?"

"Do everything" means different things to different families. In our case, the family explains that "do everything" means "do that thing you are trying to get me to agree not to do. Do CPR." In other clinical conditions, it may mean do hemodialysis, do more chemotherapy, do intubate my child again, and so on. Or do not abandon my child. Do not stop aggressively responding to changes in his clinical condition. The answer to the question of what "do everything" means to a family, whatever it is, allows you to focus on the specific meaning of "do everything" for *this* family. Do they have an experience of a family member receiving dialysis? Have they had a family member who felt abandoned by the medical team after agreeing to a DNR order? What does further chemotherapy or forgoing chemotherapy signify to them? Does forgoing cardiopulmonary resuscitation (CPR) signify giving up on their child? Does agreeing to limitations of care mean to them that they are killing their child? Understanding what "do everything" means to an individual family is an important part of developing the next steps in your plan of care. But what if, despite your best efforts, the parent(s) simply will not permit discussion of limitations of care, as in our case?

- "What do you feel you need to do to be a good parent to your child in this situation?"

Asking about what makes someone a "good parent" in their own eyes may be helpful in understanding why the parent is making the decisions he or she is making. Clinicians can use the parent's answer(s) to discuss how the clinical team may best support the parent in meeting his or her personal needs. As Feudtner et al. (2015) stated,

> Clinicians could then focus on the individual parent's answer, discussing how the clinical team can support the parent's specific aspirations, providing affirmative praise and compassionate reassurance when parents express fears that they may be failing to be, on the terms they have defined, a good parent. Furthermore, since parents may embrace a set of duties that point in different and potentially incompatible directions regarding the best plan of care, clinicians can become more aware of the tensions that parents feel while attempting to live up to apparently conflicting obligations, and then partner with parents to sort through and consider the various duties that they feel should guide their conduct. (p. 46)

MALADAPTIVE COPING AND LIMITED RESUSCITATION

In the face of a medical tragedy, some patients and families develop maladaptive coping. It has been argued that when families cannot or will not engage in discussions regarding end-of-life decision-making, a more paternalistic approach is warranted. This takes decision-making out of the hands of the family. Phrases such as "When his heart stops beating, we will not do CPR because his body is too sick to survive" may be used. This allows the family the opportunity to engage in passive nondissent, or listening to the provider but not objecting to the medical decision being made. In these situations, a unilateral DNR order—one that is instituted by the medical team due to the physiologic futility of active resuscitative measures—is ethical and appropriate if it is legal where you practice. However, some families will object when told that the team is not going to perform CPR. When this happens, some have argued that with family consent, a limited code may be the best option to assist with family coping following the death of their loved one. For a family who believes they need to know they tried "everything" to prevent their child's death, and "everything" in their minds includes CPR at end of life, a limited code may be the least bad option. However, this should only be done with a family's full understanding:

> We hear that performing CPR means you are giving your son every chance to survive, and that is important to you. And you have heard us that we do not think CPR will be helpful to your child given how sick his body is. When his heart stops beating, we will perform three rounds of CPR. If it does not work to restart your son's heart, we will stop. But we promise we will try.

This type of limited code—providing true, effective CPR but for a time-limited period—is ethically acceptable, but it can cause significant moral distress for providers. Moral distress occurs when practitioners know the ethically correct action to take (in this case, no CPR) but feel powerless to take that action (such as a provider who was not a part of the meeting where the team agreed to trial three rounds of CPR and does not agree with the plan of care). However, this type of code shows respect for the patient and family's values while limiting harm to the child.

In addition to the steps described previously, a formal ethics consult may also be helpful. Family requests for nonbeneficial treatment are common. Many physicians are willing to provide nonbeneficial treatment for a short period of time (time-limited trial) to show a family that the treatment did not achieve their stated goals. However, the American Medical Association (2016) is clear that physicians are not required to offer or to provide interventions that, in their best medical judgement, cannot reasonably be expected to yield the intended clinical benefit or achieve agreed-on goals for care. Respecting patient autonomy does not mean that patients should receive specific interventions simply because they (or their surrogates) request them.

An ethics consultation provides a third party to listen and hear the concerns of the family and the medical team and to discuss requests for nonbeneficial treatment. Even in situations in which an ethics committee suggests that a family's request for nonbeneficial treatment, such as CPR, should be honored based on the treatment's ability to honor goals of care ("We want to go down fighting!"), having a third party comment can help decrease provider moral distress.

KEY POINTS TO REMEMBER

- When a family asks you to "do everything," do not make assumptions about what that means. It is important to explore what "do everything" means to each, individual family because meanings may differ.
- Addressing goals of care is important when a child is facing end of life and the family is facing important medical decisions.
- There may be times when aggressive care at end of life is ethically acceptable, even if it may be morally distressing to providers, if it helps meet patient or family goals of care. Other times, palliative paternalism may be more appropriate.

Further Reading

American Medical Association. *Code of Medical Ethics, Annotated and Current Opinions*. Chicago, IL: American Medical Association; 2016.

Feudtner C, Morrison W. The darkening veil of "do everything." *Arch Pediatr Adolesc Med*. 2012;166(8):694–695.

Feudtner C, Walter JK, Faerber JA, et al. Good-parent beliefs of parents of seriously ill children. *JAMA Pediatr*. 2015;169(1):39–47.

Lantos JD, Meadow WL. Should the "slow code" be resuscitated? *Am J Bioeth*. 2011;11(11):8–12.

Macauley B. *Ethics in Palliative Care: A Complete Guide.* New York, NY: Oxford University Press; 2018.

Mercurio MR, Murray PD, Gross I. Unilateral pediatric "do not attempt resuscitation" orders: The pros, the cons, and a proposed approach. *Pediatrics.* 2014;133(Suppl 1):S37–S43.

Roeland E, Cain J, Onderdonk C, Kerr K, Mitchell W, Thornberry K. When open-ended questions don't work: The role of palliative paternalism in difficult medical decisions. *J Palliat Med.* 2014;17(4):415–420.

9 I Won't Let You!

Elissa G. Miller

You are caring for a 9-year-old with end-stage osteosarcoma. He has metastatic lung disease with dyspnea at rest. He also complains of chest wall pain and frequently asks for more medication. His parents, however, believe that he "doesn't need any more pain medication" and decline opioid dose escalation. You visit him and see him grimacing and crying after coughing and clutching his chest when transferring to the bedside commode. Because of both the child's requests and your clinical assessment, you believe an increase in the patient's pain medications is clinically indicated. His parents remain insistent that they will not allow their son to be on any more pain medications. A few hours later, his nurse calls you and tells you she is "going to call an ethics consult" because "I can't stand seeing him suffer and his parents won't let us treat his pain."

What do you do now?

CONFLICTS BETWEEN THE MEDICAL TEAM AND THE FAMILY

Conflicts between the medical team and the patient or patient's family arise commonly in clinical care. However, these conflicts are often most distressing when they are regarding end-of-life care, even more so when the dying patient is a child. Providers and families may disagree about, among other issues, a patient's prognosis, the use of life-sustaining medical treatment (LSMT), or, as in our case, the treatment plan.

It is not uncommon for families to disagree with providers regarding patient prognosis:

> I hear you, doc, but a few years ago the doctor told my uncle he had 6 months left to live. They put him on hospice and everything. But he's still alive and they kicked him off hospice, he was doing so well! So, I hear what you're saying, but I just don't think it's true.

By partnering with the family, stating, for example,

> I hear you, as well. And I've had situations where I was wrong in the past. I hope this is one of them, but only time will tell. I'd like to hope for the best while also still planning for the worst. Can we do that together?

families may be willing to plan as if the doctors are correct while still holding hope that the physicians' stated prognosis is wrong.

The decision to use or forgo LSMT can be emotionally difficult for patients, families, and providers. Some families believe that if they do not "try" LSMT, they are "killing" their child. Other families choose to forgo LSMT in favor of higher quality time with their child, knowing that they may have a shorter quantity of time. Still other families select a time-limited trial of LSMT to determine if it can achieve their goals of care. Conflicts between the medical team and the family arise when the medical team recommends for or against the use of a particular LSMT modality, and the family insists on the opposite. Examples of this include cardiopulmonary resuscitation, hemodialysis, intubation, and mechanical ventilation. Conflicts may also arise when a child is already being supported by significant LSMT, such as extracorporeal membrane oxygenation or a ventricular assist device, which may need to be discontinued. When conflict arises, it is important to determine if initiating, continuing, or discontinuing a particular LSMT modality would be beneficial in meeting the family's goals of care or would be nonbeneficial. For example, a family asking for endotracheal intubation for a child dying of cancer with metastases to the lungs may be able to express that they know their child cannot survive the cancer "but his grandmother is arriving tomorrow and we just want her to get here to be able to say goodbye." In such a situation, the time-limited nature of the LSMT makes providers much more willing to honor the family request. In other situations, such as a family who refuses to believe that their child with end-stage cancer is truly dying, that same LSMT may be viewed as prolonging a child's suffering and may cause significant distress among providers. In such situations, family meetings with palliative care and/or an ethics consultation may be helpful for both the care team and the family as they sort through determining the right approach for their child.

Finally, as in our case, conflicts regarding the treatment plan are not uncommon. Families often request chemotherapy past the point at which providers believe it will be beneficial to the patient and is only helping the family feel like they are "doing something." Families may also request more pain medication than a provider believes is necessary, or they may, as in our case, prevent adequate pain medication from being administered. In such situations, the conflict is often over the perceived best interest of the child. The care team believes that increased doses of pain medication are in the patient's best interest, whereas the family believes that lower doses of pain medication are in his best interest. Why does the family feel this way? What are their goals for the time their son has left? Incorporating the palliative care interdisciplinary team to talk with the family and explore the reason behind their refusal often helps in conflicts regarding treatment plans. Do they have family, religious, or cultural beliefs regarding the recommended treatment or their preferred treatment? Have they had a past experience with a family member in a similar situation? Do they believe a myth about the treatment you are recommending, and can you resolve the conflict through discussion and understanding?

Frequently in conflict resolution, providers may elicit strong emotions from the patient or family. The NURSE mnemonic is a helpful tool for handling such situations (Table 9.1).

Attentive, active listening may be most helpful in resolving family–provider conflicts because much of these conflicts arise from miscommunication.

TABLE 9.1 NURSE Mnemonic: Statements for Articulating Empathy

	Example	Notes
Naming	"It sounds like you are frustrated"	In general, turn down the intensity a notch when you name the emotion
Understanding	"This helps me understand what you are thinking"	Think of this as another kind of acknowledgment but stop short of suggesting you understand everything (you don't)
Respecting	"I can see you have really been trying to follow our instructions"	Remember that praise also fits in here eg "I think you have done a great job with this"
Supporting	"I will do my best to make sure you have what you need"	Making this kind of commitment is a powerful statement
Exploring	"Could you say more about what you mean when you say that . . ."	Asking a focused question prevents this from seeming too obvious

Source: Reprinted with permission. Copyright VitalTalk 2019.

Accordingly, you meet with your patient's family along with your palliative care team social worker. The family is tearful and tells you about the patient's grandmother, who died within a few days of initiating morphine for treatment of end-stage chronic obstructive pulmonary disease. They tell you that they are worried that increasing their son's pain medication will "kill him like it did his grandmother." You respond to the fear that the family is expressing and let them know you understand their concerns. You talk with them about other families with similar fears and talk honestly about their son's prognosis. They understand that you think he has days to weeks left to live regardless of the pain medication that is used, but that helping him be more comfortable may give him more time that will also be better quality time. His parents agree to small increases in their son's pain medication as needed. Within 24 hours, you are able to get their son much more comfortable. He has some increased sleepiness but is happier and smiles more when he is awake. His parents express relief that their son is able to enjoy the time he has left.

KEY POINTS TO REMEMBER

- Conflicts between the family and medical team arise frequently in the care of dying children.
- Using the palliative care interdisciplinary team to work with families may be sufficient to resolve the conflict. Other times, an ethics consult may be helpful if conflicts persist.
- Using the NURSE mnemonic to respond to highly charged emotional situations can be helpful.

Further Reading

Feudtner C. Collaborative communication in pediatric palliative care: A foundation for problem-solving and decision-making. *Pediatr Clin North Am.* 2007;54(5):583–607, ix.

VitalTalk. Retrieved June 7, 2019, from https://www.vitaltalk.org

Wolfe J, Hinds P, Sourkes B. *Textbook of Interdisciplinary Pediatric Palliative Care.* Philadelphia, PA: Elsevier; 2011.

10 Time to Stop

Elissa G. Miller

You are caring for a child who develops disseminated mycobacterium infection following renal transplant. He has worsening graft function of unclear etiology, and during an episode of sepsis, he is placed back on continuous renal replacement therapy (RRT) in the intensive care unit. After many weeks without return of kidney function, the team begins to discuss options for this patient. Acknowledging that he is not currently eligible for re-transplant due to active infection, his options are to transition to long-term RRT (intermittent hemodialysis or peritoneal dialysis) as destination therapy or bridge to transplant many months in the future or to discontinue RRT and provide comfort care. When you approach his parents, they tell you they "promised him he would never have to live on hemodialysis again and we will not break our promise. If you're telling us that comfort care is the only other option, I guess that's what we choose."

What do you do now?

WITHDRAWAL OF LIFE-SUSTAINING TECHNOLOGIES

Withdrawal of life-sustaining medical technologies (LSMTs) occurs commonly among patients with advanced illness. In a recent study, more than 40% of pediatric patients who died in a children's hospital died following withdrawal of LSMTs and an additional 25% following nonescalation of technology. LSMTs include enteral tube feeds, parenteral fluids and nutrition, medical devices to assist respiration, cardiopulmonary resuscitation, blood transfusions, major surgery, and antibiotics. The American Academy of Pediatrics supports withholding and withdrawing LSMTs in clinically appropriate situations, and pediatric neonatal and critical care providers are quite experienced at withholding or withdrawing intubation, mechanical ventilation, and cardiopulmonary resuscitation. However, withholding and withdrawing other medical technologies is much less common, especially in pediatrics. Various technologies that may be withdrawn are described in Table 10.1.

TABLE 10.1 **Life-Sustaining Medical Technologies That May Be Withheld or Withdrawn**

Medical Technology	Common Reasons for Withdrawal	Unique Aspects of Withdrawal
Mechanical ventilation, including noninvasive mechanical ventilation	Following devastating brain injury Due to worsening lung disease that can no longer be sustained without invasive mechanical ventilation for a family who wishes to forgo recurrent intubation and/or tracheostomy Due to worsening lung disease that can no longer be sustained without intensive care unit-level care regardless of tracheostomy status	Prognosis after withdrawal depends on both lung disease and brain disease. A patient with very sick lungs and high ventilator settings may die in minutes. A patient with a very sick brain and little or no drive to breathe may also die in minutes despite low ventilator settings and relatively healthy lungs. A patient with moderately sick lungs or a moderately injured brain may live hours to days or longer following withdrawal of mechanical ventilation.

TABLE 10.1 **Continued**

Medical Technology	Common Reasons for Withdrawal	Unique Aspects of Withdrawal
ECMO	Failed attempts at weaning ECMO despite an adequate treatment course Circuit problems such as worsening clots that are preventing the circuit from functioning appropriately Uncontrolled bleeding Family request to stop the treatment regardless of its likelihood of success	Patients often die within minutes following ECMO withdrawal due the critical nature of their illness. Families often cannot hold their child until after ECMO cannulas have been clamped and the circuit discontinued.
VAD	When heart transplantation is not an option and the VAD is causing pain and/or prolonging patient suffering	VADs are often started as a bridge to heart transplant or bridge to decision regarding heart transplant. If it is determined that the patient is not eligible for heart transplant, a VAD may help the patient live longer with a good quality of life. However, as heart failure progresses, symptoms worsen and the VAD may prolong pain and suffering.
Pacemaker/AICD	The patient is dying and the pacemaker or AICD are prolonging patient suffering	Pacemakers and AICDs are commonly used devices in adult care but rarely in pediatric care. However both are acceptable to discontinue if they are no longer helping to achieve goals of care or at end of life.

(*continued*)

TABLE 10.1 **Continued**

Medical Technology	Common Reasons for Withdrawal	Unique Aspects of Withdrawal
Tube feeds	Intestinal failure/feed intolerance causing pain and suffering When tube feeds are the only LSMT and they are artificially prolonging a patient's dying process	Withdrawal of medically administered nutrition may be emotionally difficult for families and staff because they view this as "starving" the child. However patients who are awake and alert at the time of stopping tube feeds report minimal discomfort.
Parenteral nutrition	Worsening kidney function where giving parenteral fluid causes fluid to leak into the patient's third spaces and cause pain and worsening patient suffering When parenteral nutrition is the only LSMT and it is artificially prolonging a patient's dying process or prolonging poor quality of life	This may be emotionally difficult for families unless they can clearly see the sequelae of fluid buildup.
RRT, including peritoneal dialysis, hemodialysis, and continuous veno-venous hemofiltration	Patient or family chooses not to continue treatment Patient or family chooses not to initiate treatment	Prognosis may be significantly longer than patient or family realize—7–10 days after discontinuation of chronic RRT, longer if family declines to initiate treatment depending on the clinical scenario (chronic vs. acute renal failure).

TABLE 10.1 **Continued**

Medical Technology	Common Reasons for Withdrawal	Unique Aspects of Withdrawal
Antibiotics	Smoldering infection that is causing suffering but without a realistic chance for cure Infection with multiple comorbid illnesses and antibiotics will prolong or worsen patient's suffering	Staff often worry about worsening pain with untreated infection. Some infections may be painful (e.g., urinary tract infection) and therefore within patient goals of care to treat, whereas others (e.g., endocarditis) are typically painless until tissue ischemia develops.
Blood transfusions	End-stage leukemia with blast crisis Patient older than age 18 years with religious objection to blood transfusion	Outside of end-stage leukemia, this is rarely done in pediatric palliative care because it is often viewed as a benign therapy that improves symptoms for patients with anemia. However, as patients near end of life, issues with third spacing may occur with volume administration, causing teams to re-evaluate this therapy. Difficulty transporting patients to and from a health care facility to receive the transition may become an issue as well.

AICD, automatic implantable cardioverter–defibrillator; ECMO, extracorporeal membrane oxygenation; LSMT, life-sustaining medical technology; RRT, renal replacement therapy; VAD, ventricular assist device.

ANTICIPATORY GUIDANCE

Prior to withdrawing any LSMT, it is important to provide anticipatory guidance to the family. What physical signs and symptoms should they expect to see? Advise them on expected color change and breathing changes. Discussing medications and symptom management associated with these changes is also helpful for many families. Including prognosis, as best you can, helps families know how much time they will have with their loved one after the technology is withdrawn and helps them plan who they want to have in the room at the time of withdrawal (Box 10.1). Including some uncertainty in your prognosis is also important because patients sometimes die faster or live longer than expected.

STAFF SUPPORT

Following a family's decision to withdraw LSMT, it is important to assess hospital staff feelings about the family decision. Are they relieved by the family's decision? Or upset and distressed by it? Relief may predominate when staff had been worried that a family would put their child through significant medical intervention despite a known outcome (e.g., intubation and mechanical ventilation in the setting of end-stage cancer). However, distress may predominate if the staff are not familiar with withdrawal of a particular technology or if they have their own moral and emotional judgments about withdrawing a particular technology, such as tube feeds. Working with staff who are distressed is an important role of the palliative care team. Helping them understand the family's rationale behind

---

BOX 10.1 **Increments for Patient Prognosis**

Seconds to minutes
Minutes to hours
Hours to days
Days to weeks
Weeks to months
Months to years

---

their decision, the ethics of the decision, and the American Academy of Pediatrics' position on the decision may be beneficial. Some staff may believe an ethics consult is required before the technology can be withdrawn. This should be honored although, it is hoped, without upsetting the family and causing them to second-guess their decision. Last, staff members who remain distressed or who have moral objections to participating in the care plan the family has chosen should be reminded that any staff member may recuse him- or herself from the care of any patient as long as a colleague is willing to assume care of that patient.

UNIQUE CIRCUMSTANCES

Several unique circumstances, outside of the rarely withdrawn medical technologies previously discussed, may cause significant provider distress, including the following:

- A patient is awake and cognitively intact and requesting LSMT withdrawal, such as a patient with muscular dystrophy who wants to stop his ventilator because of poor quality of life, or a child in the intensive care unit who is intubated on high ventilator settings, but awake and looking around. Discontinuing LSMT when patients are awake and alert or actively sedating an awake patient prior to LSMT withdrawal may cause significant provider distress.
- Some families are willing to withdraw some technologies but not others—for example, they are willing to discontinue inotropic blood pressure support but unwilling to stop mechanical ventilation. Others have declined further aggressive intervention but are unwilling to de-escalate, such as a family who has declined tracheostomy but who is still hoping for successful extubation with full-aggressive goals of care.
- A patient is dying slowly but has no LSMT to withdraw. Voluntary cessation of eating and drinking is an uncommon but reasonable path that adults with terminal illness may choose for end-of-life care. However, more often for a patient with no LSMT to withdraw, we discuss forgoing technologies that would prolong the patient's suffering.

All of these situations are rare in pediatrics, so they may require increased family and staff support if they occur. Also, it is important to choose your words carefully: We never withdraw *care*. We withdraw medical technology. We care for our patients until the end, and we care for their families even after our patients have died. For the patient and family in our case, the family decided to celebrate their son's life with a family party. Following the party, the team discontinued his RRT. He remained awake and alert for a few days, taking sips of clears but not eating. He became increasingly sleepy with worsening uremia until finally he was comatose. He died peacefully, surrounded by his family, 12 days after his RRT was discontinued. Although initially uncomfortable with the plan of care, staff were relieved that his death was peaceful.

> **KEY POINTS TO REMEMBER**
>
> - Withdrawal of LSMTs is common but very variable depending on the clinical condition.
> - Providing good anticipatory guidance prior to technology withdrawal is important so families can be prepared and know what to expect.
> - Providers may feel relieved by a family's choice to discontinue LSMT or may feel distressed. Providers with significant distress may recuse themselves from the care of that patient as long as a colleague is available to assume care.

Further Reading

Diekema DS, Botkin JR; Committee on Bioethics. Clinical report—Forgoing medically provided nutrition and hydration in children. *Pediatrics*. 2009;124(2):813–822.

Trowbridge A, Walter JK, McConathey E, Morrison W, Feudtner C. Modes of death within a children's hospital. *Pediatrics*. 2018;142(4):e20174182.

Weise KL, Okun AL, Carter BS, Christian CW. Guidance on forgoing life-sustaining medical treatment. *Pediatrics*. 2017;140(3):e20171905.

11   Is She Dying?

Elissa G. Miller

You are caring for an infant with metachromatic
leukodystrophy who is at home on hospice. She has
recently had no periods of alertness, and her parents
are limiting her gastric tube feeds to water due to
severe arching and pain with formula. Her breathing
remains regular, but her urine output is decreasing
and her parents are wondering, "How much time does
she have left?"

What do you do now?

CARE OF THE ACTIVELY DYING CHILD

When answering a question such as the one in our case, providers should keep the following in mind:

- Honesty
- Uncertainty

Families who are asking how much time they have left want to know, to the best of our ability, so they can plan accordingly. Whether it is to savor the time left, to call friends and family in for final goodbyes, or to know when a person's suffering is going to end, families ask because they genuinely want to know. We therefore owe it to them to be as honest and as accurate as possible. Answering with time frames is most common and recommended in palliative care (Box 11.1).

This also leaves room for the inherent uncertainty that exists, especially in prognosticating for pediatric patients whose organs are at the beginning of their typical lifespan and may continue to function beyond our expected time frame even in the setting of advanced disease.

As a child is dying, in addition to knowing expected time course, families should be offered anticipatory guidance about expected changes in the body and how we intend to work to keep their child comfortable during that time. When discussing end-of-life changes with families, we commonly review the following: breathing, vital signs, fluid status/urine output, feed tolerance, skin color, and agitation/restlessness.

BOX 11.1 **Increments for Patient Prognosis**

Seconds to minutes
Minutes to hours
Hours to days
Days to weeks
Weeks to months
Months to years

Breathing

Families can expect their child to have breathing changes as he or she is dying. Changes include shallow breathing; Cheyne–Stokes respirations; agonal breathing; and long, apneic pauses. Explaining breathing changes in words families understand, such as "gasping" and "pauses in breathing," is important. Children with pulmonary involvement of their disease process, such as advanced lung disease, heart disease with pulmonary edema, or cancer with pulmonary lesions, may have been experiencing dyspnea for some time. If the child is able to self-report, dyspnea should be treated aggressively to ensure comfort at end of life. For those who cannot self-report or who are no longer conscious and able to report, discomfort should be assessed by watching the child's body and facial expression. Any furrowing of the brow, crying, arching, flexing, or other signs of discomfort may be due to dyspnea or air hunger. This should be treated with as-needed opioid, commonly sublingual morphine. Any signs of agitation from difficulty breathing may also be managed with benzodiazepines, commonly lorazepam.

Near the end of life, children may have a buildup of secretions in the oropharynx that creates noisy breathing commonly referred to as a "death rattle." Letting families know that this is common is important. It is also important to inform them that it is not typically distressing to the patient, but suctioning to try to remove the secretions and eliminate the rattle can be distressing, so that is typically not done. We use anticholinergic agents, such as glycopyrrolate, sublingual atropine drops, atrovent puffs delivered directly to the oral mucosa, scopolamine, or hyoscyamine to minimize oral secretions and improve patient comfort. However, evidence regarding the effectiveness of these medications at decreasing noisy breathing from terminal secretions is unclear.

Vital Signs

As death becomes imminent, certain vital sign changes are expected. Commonly, children develop tachycardia due to depleted intravascular volume. Hypotension is typically a late finding and may be indicative that the child has reached the final stages of dying. Although we sometimes monitor vital signs at end of life, the only vital sign we typically respond to is fever. For a number of reasons, children may develop fevers as they are dying: Neoplastic fever and fever due to infection or atelectasis are common. Fever is typically treated with antipyretics and wet cloths to the face to prevent discomfort.

Fluid Status/Urine Output

As part of the dying process, people typically have decreasing oral intake that is progressive over time. As a result, pre-renal azotemia develops and urine output decreases. The ability to urinate spontaneously may also be affected as patients use opioids for management of air hunger, which may cause urinary retention. Urinary retention can be a source of significant discomfort for a dying patient. If this is suspected, intermittent urinary catheterization or indwelling Foley catheter placement is recommended to improve patient comfort. For patients receiving parenteral fluids or nutrition, the body's ability to handle those fluids decreases as renal function worsens, resulting in increased third spacing. Third spacing may be a source of significant discomfort as pulmonary edema, ascites, and extremity edema worsen. Minimizing parenteral fluids at end of life improves patient comfort while the patient is dying from the underlying disease process.

Feed Tolerance

Patients who are fed via feeding tube prior to the end of life will begin to show increasing feed intolerance. This is due to the shunting of blood away from the gastrointestinal tract and to the vital organs needed to maintain life. As a result, feeds may become painful to the patient and often need to be decreased or discontinued entirely. As with fluid status, the aim is to ensure comfort as the patient is dying from the underlying disease process.

Skin Color

Patients may show mottling of the skin on the extremities that waxes and wanes. However, once the extremities and trunk are mottled, this typically indicates that end of life is approaching. Informing families that children with lighter skin will have color changes, including a bluish/gray appearance, is important. Children with darker skin tones will show color changes most notably in the oropharynx and on the palms and soles. Skin changes similar to lividity—a reddish- to bluish-purple discoloration of the skin that is due to the settling and pooling of blood most typically seen following death—may develop for patients who are maintained on aggressive, life-sustaining medical treatments throughout the dying process, especially those with multiple organ system failure.

Agitation/Restlessness

Patients may exhibit agitation, restlessness, or confusion while they are dying. Agitation may be managed with benzodiazepines. However, the patient should be evaluated for delirium. If the care team suspects delirium, treating the underlying cause may or may not be possible. Therefore, treatment with antipsychotic medications is recommended. Hospice teams commonly describe terminal delirium that precedes death by hours to days, although the time frame in pediatrics is not as well established.

LOCATION OF DYING

Ideally, end-of-life care should occur in the location of the patient's or family's choosing. Common choices include at home with hospice, inpatient hospice, inpatient acute care, inpatient intensive care, or at a long-term care facility. Many families choose to be home for their child's end-of-life care. However, some worry about caring for their child at home as their child is dying. In such situations, inpatient pediatric hospice is the preferred option, but it is not always available. When inpatient pediatric hospice is not available, families may choose to receive hospice-like comfort care in an inpatient, acute care setting. Common reasons for choosing to receive comfort care in the hospital include if physical care of their child is difficult and requires multiple caregivers, if parents are divorced and prefer a neutral setting, or merely because the family feels more comfortable knowing a nurse is just down the hall. We do our best to honor the patient's and family's preferred location for end-of-life care. This includes supporting death in the intensive care unit (ICU) for families who want aggressive medical intervention at the end of their child's life if the child has a progressive disease or for those for whom an acute illness or trauma led to ICU care and ultimately withdrawal of life-sustaining medical therapies.

Conversely, some families may feel "stuck" in the ICU, and offering home terminal extubation, depending on the patient's clinical condition and the resources of the local palliative care team, can help get them out of the ICU for end-of-life care.

KEY POINTS TO REMEMBER

- Families may want to know their child's prognosis as end of life approaches. Answering with honesty while leaving room for uncertainty is important.
- Children experience a number of physical changes as death approaches. Families deserve anticipatory guidance so they know what to expect.
- Pediatric palliative care teams do their best to honor a family's preferred location for end-of-life care.

Further Reading

Harlos M. The terminal phase. In: Hanks G, et al., eds. *Oxford Textbook of Palliative Medicine* (2th ed.). New York, NY: Oxford University Press; 2010:1549–1559.

Wolfe, J. Easing distress when death is near. In: Wolfe J, ed. *Textbook of Interdisciplinary Pediatric Palliative Care*. Philadelphia, PA: Elsevier; 2011:368–384.

12 Stuck on Life Support

Elissa G. Miller

You have been caring for a 12-year-old patient
with severe mitochondrial cytopathy. He has
total intestinal failure and is dependent on total
parenteral nutrition. He also has chronic respiratory
failure and is dependent on noninvasive, positive
pressure ventilation (NIPPV) for 18 hours per day. His
pulmonologist calls you because the patient's parents
are asking about tracheostomy, yet your colleague
believes that this patient has a poor quality of life and
is "stuck" on machines. She does not want to make
his condition "worse" by putting him on a ventilator.

What do you do now?

ADVANCING TECHNOLOGY, NOW WHAT?

Medically complex pediatric patients are becoming increasingly more technology dependent. Parents in online communities share details of their child's medical care, making today's parents more connected than ever before. This sometimes leads parents to inquire about medical interventions they may have learned about from another parent whose child has the same disease. Technology such as gastric and jejunal feeding tubes, tracheostomy, ventricular assist device (VAD), and total parenteral nutrition are all discussed by parents of children with complex chronic conditions (CCCs). Providers must therefore be prepared to discuss medical technology options with their patients. The following are common questions that providers need to weigh:

- Is this technology medically indicated for this patient?
- Will this technology meet the family's goals of care?
- Will the benefits of this technology to this child outweigh the burdens?

In our case, we know that the pulmonologist believes the patient has a poor quality of life, but what do his parents think? What about the patient himself? If his parents assess that he has a poor quality of life *due to* his NIPPV, could tracheostomy possibly improve his quality of life? What if his parents assess that he has a good quality of life but he finds the NIPPV mask to be uncomfortable? Then perhaps tracheostomy could help maintain his good quality of life while improving comfort. However, if his parents believe he has a poor quality of life unrelated to his respiratory status or NIPPV, then tracheostomy is unlikely to improve his quality of life and may prolong his suffering. This, however, is not a decision the provider can make by him- or herself. This must be a discussion with the family for any technology that is medically indicated.

The benefits and burdens of a technology also must be discussed with the family. For some families, the risk of line infections and sepsis makes a technology such as home parenteral nutrition too burdensome. For others, the freedom from tube feeds that cause pain and suffering makes the risk of line infection worth the benefit of decreasing their child's suffering. Families may choose to forgo tracheostomy due to the risk that their child will not be able to talk—a shorter life with improved quality means more to them than a longer life with decreased quality. A teenager with advanced heart failure may decline VAD if he or she does not want to live connected to machines. Because some patients who initially do not want to live connected to machines may change their minds after thinking about the options and/or as their disease progresses, decisions about technology dependence and goals of care should be re-addressed regularly.

WHAT TO DISCUSS WITH FAMILIES BEFORE STARTING A NEW MEDICAL TECHNOLOGY

Prior to deciding about a new technology, families want pre- and post-decision support. Extrapolating from data on families following tracheostomy decision, they want to have the fullest understanding of possible effects of tracheostomy before it is placed and want counseling on the effects of tracheostomy on their child's and family's physical and emotional health. They want to be educated fully that respiratory issues may continue even with tracheostomy. Parents retrospectively voice frustration that quality of life was not adequately discussed prior to tracheostomy and there was too great a focus solely on survival. One study showed that only 19% of the time was foregoing tracheostomy discussed, despite 60% of the patients in the study requiring positive pressure ventilation following tracheostomy placement. Parents want their child to be physically comfortable, happy, and to maximally achieve within his or her capacity. They also need and want anticipatory guidance prior to placement of advanced medical technology as well as explanations and discussion of how the technology will affect their child's quality of life and their family functioning.

HOW TECHNOLOGY-DEPENDENT CHILDREN DIE

The majority of children with CCCs die in the hospital following withholding or withdrawal of medical technology. Therefore, before starting a new technology, it is important to discuss with families under what circumstances should that same technology be stopped, knowing that stopping it means the child cannot survive. Any technology that is an option to start is also an option to discontinue if that technology changes from helping to prolong good quality time to prolonging the child's suffering. Palliative care teams discuss this often with families facing tracheostomy decision, often when their child is intubated in the intensive care unit. Families who believe they "must" proceed with tracheostomy because they "cannot pull the plug" on their child need to know that patients with chronic ventilator dependence may die in the future from acute illness despite all aggressive measures. However, it is also possible that a patient with chronic ventilator dependence may suffer a decline that would leave the patient too sick to survive outside an intensive care unit but not actively dying. In such a situation, families may have to discontinue their child's chronic ventilator. For some families, this risk is worth the life-prolonging benefit of tracheostomy. For other families, the idea that they may someday have to "pull the plug" on their loved one makes them prefer to initiate a do not intubate/do no resuscitate order so they are never put in that situation. Like the family in our case, this is better discussed in advance so families have the opportunity to plan and explore all options. Joining with medical and surgical colleagues to initiate early conversations prior to initiation or surgical placement of advanced technology can aid families in exploration of benefits/burdens and advanced care planning.

KEY POINTS TO REMEMBER

- Helping families weigh the benefits and burdens prior to initiating a new medical technology is extremely important.
- Before making the decision to initiate a new technology, families want to know as much as possible about how the patient's life will be affected after adding it.
- Any technology that is added may need to be stopped in the future, and this should be discussed prior to starting the new technology.

Further Reading

Baumgardner D. Families at risk: Quality of life in technology-dependent children and their families. *The Exceptional Parent*; March 1999.

Cohen E, Kuo DZ, Agrawal R., et al. Children with medical complexity: An emerging population for clinical and research initiatives. *Pediatrics*. 2011;127(3):529–538.

DeCourcey DD, Silverman M, Oladunjoye A, Balkin EM, Wolfe J. Patterns of care at the end of life for children and young adults with life-threatening complex chronic conditions. *J Pediatr*. 2018;193:196–203.

Graf J, Montagnino B, Hueckel R, McPherson M. Pediatric tracheostomies: A recent experience from one academic center. *Pediatr Crit Care Med*. 2008;9(1):96–100.

Hopkins C, Whetstone S, Foster T, Blaney S, Morrison G. The impact of paediatric tracheostomy on both patient and parent. *Int J Pediatr Otorhinolaryngol*. 2009;73:15–20.

13 How Do We Go Back to Work Now?

Lindsay B. Ragsdale

You are called frantically to the bedside of a 6-year-old child in the pediatric intensive care unit (ICU) who arrested and received cardiopulmonary resuscitation (CPR) for 45 minutes. She did not respond to CPR and was just pronounced dead. Some of the members of the ICU team are crying in the hallway, and one ICU physician is angry and just stormed out of the ICU. The patient was much beloved by the hospital staff as she was admitted often, and her parents did a great job taking care of her. She has had many admissions for her short gut syndrome and central line infections. She has arrested in the past but has always been able to return to baseline and go home. She has not needed to be admitted for the past year, and everyone thought she was doing much better. The chaplain is at the bedside taking care of grieving parents. The staff is glad that you are there to provide support to them. They ask you how they can return to care for the ICU full of patients.

What do you do now?

DEBRIEFING AFTER SIGNIFICANT PATIENT EVENT

Medical care can be unpredictable and erratic at times due to fluctuating clinical status; emergencies; medical errors; limitations of medical science; and the emotions of patients, families, and staff that are associated with illness. Even with improved processes and quality initiatives, there are times when patient outcomes are not what we are hoping for due to many complex factors. Medical professionals are present during these very intense patient experiences which can leave an emotional residue that can accumulate over time, adding to job dissatisfaction, psychological distress, and burnout. Debriefing after a significant patient event can help provide a time for medical staff to discuss the event, talk about their emotions, enhance teamwork, and improve the feeling of being supported by peers. In fact, growing literature supports the fact that debriefing after a critical event can improve outcomes in subsequent critical events. Pediatric palliative care teams in many areas can help facilitate debriefings or can help train a local champion to host them. Palliative care teams are present during these critical events and have experience with maintaining resiliency while taking care of critically ill and dying patients.

A code is an example of a critical event that requires a highly functional team with clear communication combined with heightened stress levels in the providers involved. This combination has the potential to create confusion and less optimal interpersonal interactions leading to worse outcomes. These factors can weigh on providers and contribute to distress after a code. Many institutions have implemented a post code discussion, and this is becoming standard practice. This discussion allows for code members to talk about the events of the code and identify what went well and areas for improvement. The discussion also allows space to talk about the emotional impact of the code on the providers and to identify what might help them return back to patient care. The debriefing should be a non-blame environment and allow members of the code team to ask questions and learn without judgment. Some institutions use trained facilitators for these discussions, whereas others identify a specific member of the code team to initiate and facilitate the discussion. There is growing evidence that debriefing a code can improve the performance at the next code, including communication and chest compression depth. Also, these debriefs can allow providers the opportunity to honor the patient if the patient died and to reflect on their experience of the patient's death. Even in busy emergency rooms, implementing a brief post code discussion is feasible and can help support emergency room staff, who are at high risk for burnout as a group. In our case, the ICU staff are grieving the loss of their patient in different ways and struggling to find a way to return to caring for their other patients. A debrief can help bring the code team together and unpack the events and discuss them. Although a larger debrief may be helpful for the entire unit, bringing the members of the code team together during this shift will assist in addressing the acute needs of the team.

For our case, the palliative care social worker and physician suggested that they have a post code debriefing and secured a private conference room in the ICU. The code team assembled, and even the ICU physician who was angry attended after the palliative physician talked with him. The discussion was facilitated by the palliative care team, including discussions of the peri-code events, code mechanics, communication, equipment/medication availability, and decision to call the code and pronounce the patient dead. The conversation was tense and emotional at first, but as team members started talking about what went right, everyone started talking more freely. Many of the ICU nurses talked about how much the ICU physician had done to help the patient and that he had exhausted all the available resuscitative efforts. He was able to identify his feelings of failing the patient and her parents. He was supported by his ICU colleagues who share their sadness of her dying. However, during the discussion, he was able to agree that her body was so overwhelmed by sepsis that she was unable to be rescued. They identified the need for codes to be quieter so that they could hear the directions of the code leader. They also had a moment of silence to honor their patient and her bravery; they brought her parents into the moment of silence and all held hands. After the debriefing, everyone supported each other and they were able to return to the bedside of the other patients in the ICU. The debriefing took approximately 10 minutes, and the nurse managers in the ICU watched the other patients during the debriefing. The ICU physician thanked the palliative care physician for encouraging him to attend the debriefing because this allowed him to unpack the feelings of guilt and shame and not internalize them. He acknowledged that he has not done this in the past and has carried the guilt from past patient deaths with him over time. The palliative team hosted a debriefing for the entire unit at change of shift the next day and allowed a space for the ICU staff to process what happened to their patient.

Most health care providers can easily identify a code as a reason to debrief because this is a dramatic medical event. However, more subtle stressors can be an opportunity to debrief—for example, violent or aggressive behavior of a family member or staff member. One hospital hosted a debriefing after a father of a neonatal ICU patient threw a chair at a nurse when he learned about his premature daughter's intracerebral hemorrhages; fortunately, the nurse was not injured. The father was escorted out of the unit by security and had to meet with police, social workers, and the hospital legal team about the incident. The father had a history of aggressive communication, and even before this event occurred, the staff felt uncomfortable when he was in the unit. The debriefing allowed an opportunity for the staff to express their fear and worry about their safety. This was also an opportunity to discuss workplace violence, available support, and security measures. With the help of a nurse manager and social worker, they were able to identify security strategies and boundaries for their unit moving forward. This allowed many nurses in this unit to feel they were being heard and to explore their feelings of safety at work.

Medical error disclosure can be a time of intensity and stress for providers, patients, and family. As medicine strives for more transparency and quality improvement initiatives, disclosures of medical errors are increasing and can contribute to global stress on a provider. Debriefing with the providers involved in medical errors can allow space to explore emotions associated with these events and to connect providers to resources such as counseling and peer support. Legal implications of a medical error can weigh heavily on a physician and can challenge the social expectations of a physician to be infallible. Some institutions hold root cause analysis meetings soon after these events to identify system or processes changes that can be implemented to avoid errors in the future. However, these might not fully address the personal distress of the providers involved, and further support or counseling may be needed.

Debriefs can be constructed in any way that is conducive to the team members involved. Evidence shows that code reviews are best done in smaller groups with just the code team involved. However, for unit-wide issues, a large debrief might be more helpful. Many institutions have been able to institute regular debriefs to discuss the effects of patient care on

TABLE 13.1 Questions to Help Facilitate a Debrief

What went right with the case?

What could be improved with this case?

How did we support the family?

How did this case make you feel?

What did you learn from this case?

What will you take with you to your next patient?

the staff and also on-demand debriefs for issues that arise in between regularly scheduled debriefs. This scheduling allows opportunities to practice regular self-reflection of staff to build self-preservation and also provides opportunities for crisis management. Table 13.1 presents examples of questions that can be used at a debrief to help stimulate conversation. Schwartz Center Rounds® have been initiated at some institutions to help medical staff and learners discuss the impact of medicine on them as individuals in a nonthreatening environment. These rounds can be an opportunity to have open discussions of challenges, stressors, and benefits of taking care of patients as a larger medical community. Some more sensitive topics may require one-on-one discussion and referrals to further counseling resources. Staff support initiatives can involve existing professionals in an institution for facilitation, including palliative care teams, chaplains, licensed clinical social workers, and psychologists.

KEY POINTS TO REMEMBER

- Post code discussions can help staff talk about their emotions related to a case.
- Post code discussions can improve outcomes in subsequent codes.
- Debriefs can be helpful for staff to unpack difficult cases and prevent distress.
- Debriefs can be used as a one-on-one discussion or as a larger unit discussion.

Further Reading

Copeland, D, Liska H. Implementation of a post-code pause: Extending post-event debriefing to include silence. *J Trauma Nurs.* 2016; 23(2): 58–64.

Fritz Z, Slowther AM, Perkins GD. Resuscitation policy should focus on the patient, not the decision. *BMJ.* 2017; 356:J813.

Hannawa AF, Beckman H, Mazor KM, Paul N, Ramsey JV. Building bridges: Future directions for medical error disclosure research. *Patient Educ Couns.* 2013;92(3):319–327.

Hughes J, Duff AJ, Puntis JWL. Using Schwartz Center Rounds to promote compassionate care in a children's hospital. *Arch Dis Child.* 2018;103(1):11–12.

Riskin A, Erez A, Foulk TA, et al. The impact of rudeness on medical team performance: A randomized trial. *Pediatrics.* 2015;136(3):487–495.

Wolfe H, Zebuhr C, Topjian AA, et al. Interdisciplinary ICU cardiac arrest debriefing improves survival outcomes. *Crit Care Med.* 2014;42(7):1688–1695.

Zebuhr C, Sutton RM, Morrison W, et al. Evaluation of quantitative debriefing after pediatric cardiac arrest. *Resuscitation* 2012;83(9):1124–1128.

14 Always Putting My Needs Last

Lindsay B. Ragsdale

You are asked to consult on a 11-month-old infant with 22q11 deletion, absence of the corpus callosum, congenital heart disease, and home tracheostomy and ventilator dependence. He has been admitted to the intensive care unit (ICU) at least 1 week per month for the past 6 months. His feeding schedule is every 3 hours during the day and night, with feeds lasting more than 1½ hours. His father works full-time during evening shifts, and his mother quit her job to stay at home and take care of their son. They do not have any family in the area because they recently moved to the area for the father's job. The mother has performed cardiopulmonary resuscitation (CPR) twice on her son during times of crisis and blames herself for his many admissions. When you ask if she has slept or eaten anything in the past 24 hours, she becomes tearful and says that her focus is on her son and her needs should always come last.

What do you do now?

CARING FOR THE CAREGIVER

As medical care for pediatric patients has become more complex, the stress and burdens on families have increased as well. The toll that this intense medical care can take on family/caregivers can be significant and can have downstream effects on health-related outcomes of the patient. There is evidence that significant stressors can affect the physical and emotional health of the caregiver and can have implications for the well-being of the caregiver in the long term, even increasing caregiver mortality risk. Emerging data also indicate that having a sick child can have deleterious effects on the parents' relationship and can increase risk of divorce or dissolution of the relationship. Palliative teams can add an additional layer of support for caregivers and perform a comprehensive needs assessment to identify potential interventions to mitigate stress points. Layering in-home nursing, respite, financial resources, counseling, and exploring meaning can help offset the challenges of intense medical care.

A caregiver assessment should occur as part of a comprehensive palliative care consult and should include evaluation of the following:

1. Basic needs of food, shelter, warmth, safety, and rest
2. Caregiver stress and exhaustion factors
3. Clarity of medical care and prognosis
4. Social and economic needs
5. Spiritual and existential issues

Once the caregiver assessment has been completed, the palliative team should create an individualized plan for supporting the caregiver. This plan might be different for each caregiver in a particular home and also will vary from family to family. Part of the unique aspect of palliative care is the ability to get to know patients and caregivers on an individual basis, and this relationship building can help refine the support for caregivers over time. Table 14.1 lists commonly used caregiver assessment tools to help identify stress points and to facilitate a conversation with the caregiver. These assessments can be used initially to pinpoint needs but also can be repeated over time to ensure that the supports put in place are helping decrease caregiver strain and stress. These assessment tools can help identify which person in the palliative care interdisciplinary team is best suited to help the caregiver with the

TABLE 14.1	**Caregiver Assessment Tools**

Parenting Stress Index (PSI) Short Form

Pediatric Inventory for Parents (PIP)

Pearlin Role Overload Measure (ROM)

Caregiver Self-Assessment Questionnaire

Caregiver Inventory (CGI)

Caregiver Burden Scale

Parenting Routines Inventory–Stress Scale

stress points. If basic necessities are the greatest need, then a social worker might be the best professional within the team to have a further discussion with the caregiver about these issues. Some parents have described feeling socially isolated and trapped at home, which exacerbates their feelings of hopelessness and depression. An assessment tool may highlight the need for respite care or for peer supports for the parents to feel less isolated. If existential concerns are the primary issue, then a chaplain may be best suited to further explore beliefs and assess for meaning, fears, hopes, guilt, and/ or forgiveness. The palliative care team should work together to help assess and support caregivers during their illness journey. For example, a chaplain may have an in-depth discussion with a parent who reveals their biggest fear for their child is shortness of breath at end of life. This fear has impacted the parent's sleep patterns and appetite because the parent is continually focusing on this fear. The chaplain can discuss this fear with the care team to help make a plan for symptom management and to reassure the parent that they will meticulously attend to their child's symptoms. The chaplain can continue to explore these worries with the parent to try to reframe the repeating worries and to minimize the impact on caregiver's health. This interdisciplinary work is integral to palliative care and should be woven throughout the care of the child and the caregiver.

Many children with complex chronic conditions can live years with intense medical care; the intensity of the care can weigh on caregivers over months and years. The care of a child with a serious illness often encompasses all domains of needs, including physical, emotional, social, spiritual, activities of daily living, financial, advocacy, nursing, coordinator of care, transporter, and communicator, in addition to the "standard parent" duties. It is foreseeable that the burden put on parents and/or caregivers is immense and constant. Helping assess or even predict the burdens for caregivers is important to managing expectations. The caregiver's expectations can change their perception of how well they are doing as a caregiver. Some caregivers have had little anticipatory guidance on the burdens of care of a medically complex child before going home for the first time. This lack of guidance can lead to the caregiver feeling guilty, inadequate, and like a failure. It has been shown that the overarching need of a parent is to feel like they are being a "good parent." We can help support this duty to be a "good parent" by thoroughly advising the caregiver on the realities of the medical care and the implications to the caregiver's daily life in all domains. It is important to assess and layer in support for caregivers when available because this can directly impact the physical and emotional health of the caregiver and the medical care the patient will receive at home.

The 11-month-old child you were asked to see has complex medical health care needs at home, including around-the-clock feeds, tracheostomy suctioning, and repositioning. During this admission, his mother is showing signs of caregiver stress. The best approach is to take some time to assess their supports at home, including physical, social, emotional, and financial support. The mother has not been taking care of her own basic needs of sleep and nutrition in lieu of her son's needs. You could frame this discussion around how well she has taken care of her son and reinforce the amazing job she has been doing taking care of the whole family (this could help address the duty to feel like a good parent). You can directly address the arrest episodes and the need for repeated admissions, which are not a result of the care the parents have been giving but, rather, a reflection of their son's condition. You can discuss your expectations for their son and what would be anticipated burdens of care long term to set reasonable expectations. You talk to your social worker on the unit to explore ways for the mother to eat dinner and have a place to rest tonight. Your assessment reveals the patient's medical care is around the clock without adequate time for the mother to sleep. You talk with your discharge planners and social workers about home nursing options for them to allow the mother adequate sleep and to simplify the medical regimen when possible.

You discover that the parents are managing the stress in different ways. The mother has signs of post-traumatic stress after having to perform CPR on her son and wishes to talk to a psychologist. The father relies heavily on his faith and is praying for his son every day and has hope for his long-term recovery. You talk with the chaplain about the father's expression of faith, and they explore further about his beliefs and hopes. The social worker discovers that their insurance allows for respite care one night a month for the parents to participate in an activity together outside of the home.

You also arrange follow up with the pediatric palliative care team because the infant has repeated admissions to the ICU and a serious illness with an unclear prognosis. The team will continue to support the parents and frequently reassess their caregiver stress levels and make adjustments as needed.

KEY POINTS TO REMEMBER

· Caregiver well-being can directly impact the health of a child with a serious illness.
· Caregiver assessment tools can help identify needs and follow stress level over time.
· Physical, spiritual, emotional, and socioeconomic domains of the caregiver's life can be impacted by caregiver responsibilities.
· Offer anticipatory guidance about the realities and burdens of care at home, and help the caregiver readjust expectations when needed.

Further Reading
Cousino M, Hazen R. Parenting stress among caregivers of children with chronic illness: A systematic review. *J Pediatr Psychol.* 2013;38(8):809–828.
Empeno J, Raming NT, Irwin SA, Nelesen RA, Lloyd LS. The Hospice Caregiver Support Project: Providing support to reduce caregiver stress. *J Palliat Med.* 2011;14(5):593–597.

Koch KD, Jones BL. Supporting parent caregivers of children with life-limiting illness. *Children.* 2018;5(7):85.

Verberne LM, Kars MC, Schouten-van Meeteren AYN, et al. Aims and tasks in parental caregiving for children receiving palliative care at home: A qualitative study. *Eur J Pediatr.* 2017;176:343–354.

Vrijmoet-Wiersma CM, van Klink JM, Kolk AM, Koopman HM, Ball LM, Maarten Egeler R. Assessment of parental psychological stress in pediatric cancer: A review. *J Pediatr Psychol.* 2008;33(7):694–706.

Symptom Management

15 My Stomach Hurts

David Flemig

You are seeing a 14-year-old female with an 18-month history of abdominal pain. The pain initially started after eating, but it has progressed to be a diffuse, constant ache, with flares of migratory postprandial cramping. She also has diarrhea and 40-pound weight loss in the past 3 months, prompting her current hospitalization. She has undergone two upper and lower endoscopies in the past 6 months, which were inconclusive and left her fearful of further interventions. The frequent pain episodes have started to make her feel anxious about eating, which is causing insomnia. It is interfering with her relationships at school, and the uncertainty of her condition is triggering distress. She has tried several different medications unsuccessfully for symptom control, including hyoscamine, simethicone, and ketorolac. During her current admission, she was started on oxycodone for acute pain, which helped. The family asks how you are planning to better control her pain.

What do you do now?

UNCONTROLLED PAIN

Pain is a subjective experience that can be attributed to a variety of sources, not all of them from underlying organic disease. It can be a presentation of psychological, spiritual, or social distress, so a comprehensive pain assessment includes discussing these domains with every patient who has uncontrolled pain.

Second, it is important to remember that treating the underlying cause of pain is the best way to reduce symptoms. Sometimes an underlying cause cannot be identified or treated; therefore, relying on good symptom control with pharmacologic and nonpharmacologic means can relieve suffering. This chapter discusses matching the appropriate medication to the various types of pain. After trialing an intervention for symptom control, it is imperative to reassess symptoms and possible side effects of therapy.

The patient in this case has several different triggers for her pain. First is her physical pain from her undiagnosed gastrointestinal illness. This physical pain has allowed for the development of psychological distress, as evidenced by her anxiety around eating, fear of procedures, and inability to sleep. She also has developed symptoms related to change in her social domain: fluctuations in her school relationships and uncertainty about her future.

All of these domains contribute to her current total pain experience and must be addressed to help completely treat her pain. Although other members of the palliative care team, such as social workers, chaplains, and psychologists, are better trained to help with the spiritual, social, and psychological aspects of pain, it is important for all palliative care providers to have a basic understanding of these pain domains to screen for their contribution to symptoms. Further discussion of these domains is outside the scope of this chapter, so the focus here is on the physical aspects of her pain.

To start an assessment of physical pain, a standardized approach can help classify the type of pain each patient is experiencing, which will thereby lead to choice of an appropriate medication and ultimately better symptom control. The assessment is limited by the developmental level of the child (see Chapter 18, this volume). Key details in a comprehensive physical pain history of a verbal patient include the following:

1. Location of pain
2. Onset, duration, fluctuation, and severity
3. Triggers and alleviating factors
4. Quality of pain (burning, sharp, or aching)
5. Radiation or referral of pain

Physical pain is a complex process, but it can roughly be classified as nociceptive pain and neuropathic pain. Nociceptive pain is caused by tissue damage triggering activation of nociceptive nerve fibers, which when activated in the skin, soft tissues, bones, or joints is classified as somatic pain. Activation of nociceptors in the visceral organs is classified as visceral pain. Somatic pain is typically localized and is exacerbated by movement, whereas visceral pain is typically more generalized and can often be experienced as referred pain to different regions of the body (e.g., right scapular pain in cholecystitis). Neuropathic pain is caused by damage to the nerves and is distributed along the path of the nerves involved. Neuropathic pain can be described as "burning," "lancinating," or "tingling," and it can present as an exaggerated response to a painful stimulus (hyperalgesia) or as pain caused by something that does not normally produce pain (allodynia). Mixed pain is a combination of nociceptive and neuropathic pain and is commonly found in cancer pain.

These classifications are helpful because each type of pain has different presenting symptoms, respond to different medications, or could be amenable to interventional procedures (if the symptoms are localized). Table 15.1 provides a breakdown of the different pain types, their characteristic symptoms, and classes of medication used for treatment.

Let's return to the case. She appears to have a component of all three types of physical pain (remember to not forget the other domains of her pain—psychological, spiritual, and social). The dull ache suggests somatic pain, whereas the cramping aspect suggests visceral pain. The pain caused after a normally nonpainful experience (allodynia)—eating—is indicative of neuropathic pain. Therefore, medications that target all three components

TABLE 15.1   **Pain Types, Their Causes, Descriptors, and Treatment Options**

Pain Type	Causes	Descriptors	Medications and Interventions
Somatic nociceptive pain	Damage to tissue of skin, soft tissue, bones, and muscles	Aching, deep, dull, sharp, and stabbing	Acetaminophen Nonsteroidal anti-inflammatory Opioids Steroids Surgery Radiation Interventional procedures
Visceral nociceptive pain	Damage to visceral organs such as intestines, stomach, liver, and pancreas	Cramping, squeezing, bloating, fullness, and gas	Acetaminophen Nonsteroidal anti-inflammatory Opioids Steroids Radiation Surgery Interventional procedures
Neuropathic pain	Injury or inflammation of nerves	Burning, electricity, numb, tingling, pins and needles, hyperalgesia, and allodynia	Gabapentinoids (gabapentin and pregabalin) Antidepressants (amitriptyline and duloxetine) Ketamine Opioids Radiation Interventional procedures

must be used. Remember, diagnosis and treatment of her underlying condition will lead to the greatest improvement in her symptoms overall, but we can try to manage her symptoms in the meantime.

When choosing a medication, there are several factors to consider:

1. What are my goals of treatment?
2. What type of pain am I dealing with?

3. Are there any patient allergies?
4. What are the risks and side effects of each medication?
5. How will I administer the medication?

The remainder of this chapter focuses on establishing treatment goals and the risks and side effects of various medications.

Often in palliative care, we are not able to fully cure a disease, so it is difficult to completely eliminate the pain that a patient experiences. This is important to remember when establishing treatment goals with patients and family members. Sometimes the goal is not to completely eliminate pain but, rather, to reach an acceptable pain level to allow the patient to perform a particular task, participate in physical therapy, or perform other activities of daily living. Clear goals can also help guide medication selection and titration.

When initiating a medication for pain, it is prudent to follow the general rule of "start low, go slow." If your patient is experiencing complex or refractory pain, consider consulting palliative care or pain management to expedite symptom control.

Next, several commonly used analgesics and their side effects are briefly discussed.

NON-OPIOIDS: ACETAMINOPHEN AND NONSTEROIDAL ANTI-INFLAMMATORY DRUGS

Acetaminophen is one of the first-line agents for the treatment of pain in children of any age, but its mechanism of action is still poorly understood. Because acetaminophen is metabolized by the liver, its use in patients with hepatic dysfunction is limited. Excessive use can also cause acute liver failure. Acetaminophen has no anti-inflammatory properties.

Nonsteroidal anti-inflammatory drugs (NSAIDs), such as ibuprofen and naproxen, work through inhibition of the cyclooxygenase enzyme, which limits the inflammatory cascade. NSAIDs may cause renal dysfunction, gastritis, or platelet dysfunction.

Use of both acetaminophen and NSAIDs may be limited by their antipyretic effects if an important component of care is monitoring the child's fever curve.

OPIOIDS

Opioids such as morphine, oxycodone, hydromorphone, methadone, and fentanyl work by binding to receptors in the central nervous system and inhibiting ascending pain pathways. Opioids can be administered in various routes, so important considerations for selection include pain severity, dose timing, and understanding universal opioid side effects.

Patients can develop tolerance to certain opioid side effects such as nausea, vomiting, dizziness, sedation, and respiratory depression. These should be anticipated and monitored closely with initiation and escalation of opioid therapy. Other side effects, such as constipation, usually do not subside with continued use and will need to be monitored closely to avoid abdominal pain and obstipation. Care should also be taken in patients with renal dysfunction because this can predispose to myoclonus due to opioids. Pruritus is most common with morphine and can be managed with antihistamines as first-line therapy. If significant side effects of opioid therapy develop, consider opioid rotation or low-dose naloxone or nalbuphine to counteract the side effects especially of pruritus and urinary retention.

ADJUVANTS

This group of medications consists of agents with a benefit of analgesia in addition to their primary use. Broadly speaking, there are antidepressants, steroids, and antiepileptics.

Antidepressants: Tricyclic Antidepressants and Selective Norepinephrine Reuptake Inhibitors

The mechanism of pain relief for antidepressants is incompletely understood. Of the tricyclic antidepressants, amitriptyline has the most analgesic evidence and is helpful for the treatment of neuropathic pain and the prevention of migraines. Its side effect profile includes sedation, anticholinergic effects, and QT prolongation, so electrocardiogram monitoring of the QT interval could be considered with initiation and dosing changes.

Duloxetine has the most evidence for pain relief of the selective norepinephrine reuptake inhibitors and can be used for musculoskeletal pain (it is particularly helpful in fibromyalgia) and neuropathic pain. There is little evidence that the selective serotonin reuptake inhibitors have any significant analgesic effect. The main side effects of duloxetine include nausea, sedation, and sexual dysfunction.

Steroids

These medications are helpful for relief of inflammation and are particularly helpful for malignant bone pain. Their main side effects include agitation, gastritis, myopathy, and reduced immunity.

Gabapentinoids

The gabapentinoids (gabapentin and pregabalin) are useful for the treatment of neuropathic pain. They are thought to bind to central nervous system receptors and inhibit the response to pain by modulating release of excitatory neurotransmitters. Their major side effects include sedation, dizziness, and lower extremity edema.

N-Methyl-d-Aspartate (NMDA) Receptor Antagonists

Ketamine can be utilized for reduction of neuropathic pain. Its mechanism of analgesia is also incompletely understood, but it is thought to occur in part through its effects on the NMDA receptors at subanesthetic doses. The main side effects include psychomimetic effects and delirium. Methadone is a long half-life opioid with NMDA receptor activity that can be useful for mixed somatic and neuropathic pain. Both Methadone and Ketamine should be prescribed only by providers comfortable with their use.

Radiation Therapy and Regional Anesthesia

Although outside the scope of this chapter, it is worth mentioning the benefits of regional anesthesia and radiation therapy for localized pain. These modalities should be chosen with the help of palliative care, anesthesia, pain, or radiation specialists.

SUMMARY

Now that we have reviewed various pharmacologic agents to treat pain, let's return to the patient. To target her somatic and visceral nociceptive pain, we recommended scheduled acetaminophen and utilizing as-needed ibuprofen and oxycodone for breakthrough pain. For her neuropathic pain, we recommended starting gabapentin. In addition to pharmacologic treatment, she started working with the social worker and psychologist to identify how other domains of pain are contributing to her suffering. This combination decreased the intensity of her chronic dull ache and also minimized the severity of her postprandial flares. Ultimately, she was started on steroids when her gastroenterologists diagnosed her with eosinophilic gastroenteritis, so this further reduced her pain from its nociceptive component.

KEY POINTS TO REMEMBER

- Pain is a complex interplay of many different domains— physical, social, spiritual, and psychological. Uncontrolled pain requires a comprehensive assessment of all these areas.
- The best way to control pain is to treat the underlying cause. Until that can be achieved, match medicines that will treat the type of pain the patient is experiencing (somatic, visceral, or nociceptive) to minimize suffering from pain.
- Reassess after any interventions, and monitor for side effects of therapy.
- Ask for help from palliative and pain specialists if your patient has refractory pain.

Further Reading

Collins JJ, Berde CB, Frost JA. Pain assessment and management. In Wolfe J, Hinds P, Sourkes B, eds. *Textbook of Interdisciplinary Pediatric Palliative Care*. Philadelphia, PA: Elsevier; 2011:284–299.

Rork JF, Berde CB, Goldstein RD. Regional anesthesia approaches to pain management in pediatric palliative care: A review of current knowledge. *J Pain Symptom Manage*. 2013;46(6):859–873.

World Health Organization. *WHO Guidelines on the Pharmacological Treatment of Persisting Pain in Children with Medical Illness*. Geneva, Switzerland: World Health Organization; 2012.

16 No Access and Still in Pain

Lindsay B. Ragsdale

You are asked to see a 10-day-old neonate who has an unrepaired gastroschisis, tracheoesophageal fistula with esophageal atresia, and a brain abnormality, with no ability to administer enteral feeds or medications. The neonate is intubated and has struggled with agitation and pain behaviors, but he was finally less agitated after starting fentanyl through a peripheral intravenous (IV) catheter. The neonatal intensive care unit (NICU) calls you back to the bedside because the neonate lost IV access and they cannot find any additional peripheral sites for an IV and the central line team is not available. They ask you how they should keep the neonate comfortable now.

What do you do now?

ROUTES OF PAIN MEDICATIONS FOR CHILDREN

Selecting a pain medication for a child should depend on many factors, including the possible routes of delivery. The most common routes of pain medication delivery are oral/per tube, sublingual, IV, subcutaneous, intranasal, rectal, inhaled, and transdermal. This chapter reviews the most common routes and helps providers match the best route with their patient's individual needs. In general, the least invasive route should be used first in pediatric patients. Table 16.1 lists common medications used for palliative symptom management that can be given by different routes.

ORAL/PER TUBE

The most common route of pain medication delivery is the oral route. It is also considered the least invasive route. However, children may find it difficult to swallow a pill even until adolescent age ranges. Young children can be taught the skill of swallowing a pill; however, learning this skill might not be worth the investment depending on the developmental level and prognosis of illness. Over-the-counter oral pill glide sprays are available in a variety of flavors to help with difficulty swallowing pills. Capsules can sometimes be broken open and the internal sprinkles can be put into a small amount of pudding, yogurt, or apple sauce if the child is old enough or developmentally able to swallow solids.

Oral medications can often be compounded into a solution or suspension and administered with an oral syringe or medication cup. Flavoring (dye, sugar, and gluten- and casein-free flavoring agents are available) can be added to the medication liquids based on their chemical compounds to create the most palatable taste. There are many online resources (e.g., http://www.flavorx.com) to match each medication with the best flavor. However, even with flavoring, some medications can be unpleasant tasting, and children may refuse to take them despite best efforts. Some young infants can have medications administered by oral syringe in the back of their mouth, and the natural swallow reflex, if neurologically intact, will help them swallow the liquid. Older children may become upset and more agitated by being forced to take liquid medications and can spit the medication or have vomiting after administering it by mouth. Most pediatric providers use a

TABLE 16.1 **Routes of Delivery of Common Palliative Medications**

Oral/Per Tube	Intravenous	Subcutaneous	Transdermal	Intranasal	Inhaled	Rectal
Acetaminophen	Acetaminophen	Morphine	Fentanyl	Fentanyl	Morphine	Acetaminophen
Ibuprofen	Ketorolac	Hydromorphone	Clonidine	Ketamine	Hydromorphone	Diazepam
Morphine	Morphine	Fentanyl		Midazolam	Fentanyl	Morphine
Hydromorphone	Hydromorphone			Dexmedetomidine		Hydromorphone
Oxycodone	Fentanyl					Promethazine
Methadone	Ketamine					Phenobarbital
Clonidine	Methadone					
Ketamine	Dexmedetomidine					
Ketorolac						

strategy to focus on alleviating pain and not cause more distress with each dose. Talk with caregivers about the child's response to taking medications in the past, and match the route with the individual child.

Immediate-acting liquid pain medications can be safely given per tube, both gastric and post-pyloric tubes. Some capsule sprinkles or crushed pills can clog feeding tubes, so ensure each medication has been cleared for feeding tube administration before prescribing. In the instance of multiple medications given per tube at once, be cognizant of the sorbitol (polyalcohol sugar commonly added to liquid medications) content of each medication because this can cause bloating, gas, and abdominal discomfort at doses of 10 g per day or more.

The challenge with oral pain medications can occur when an extended-release/sustained-release medication is needed in addition to immediate-release medications. These extended-release tablets cannot be crushed and administered in a feeding tube, and no sprinkle capsule formulations are currently on the market. If an extended-release formulation is needed, oral tablet swallowed or transdermal patches are the two most common options for pediatrics. Currently, methadone is the only long-acting opioid in a liquid formulation.

INTRAVENOUS

Intravenous administration of pain medications is often used in the acute care setting for control of acute flares or incidental pain related to procedures. For pediatric patients, finding peripheral IV access can be challenging due to the small caliber of veins and also subcutaneous fat deposition, so it is important to use the most skilled provider to place the IV catheter. Depending on the developmental age and activity level of the child, the IV catheter site may need to be reinforced and the joint softly immobilized to prevent the patient from tampering with the catheter. Using distraction and topical anesthetic agents, such as freeze spray or lidocaine creams, when obtaining access can decrease distress of the pediatric patient. Dosing of IV pain medications may need to be scheduled instead of written "as needed" to ensure adequate analgesia if patients are reluctant or unable to voice when they are in pain. For children with serious illness, IV medications may be warranted at home for a longer time frame or at end of life. Some patients may need a central line, port, or peripherally inserted central catheter (PICC) placed for long-term access and for administration of medications or fluids. These IV access catheters can be used for continuous or intermittent administration of pain medications. At end of life, many hospices will use home patient-controlled analgesic machines to safely administer doses of pain medications with basal rates and on-demand doses regulated with maximum doses.

SUBCUTANEOUS

Subcutaneous administration of pain medications can be used safely in pediatric patients, even neonates. A subcutaneous catheter can be placed in the subcutaneous space with a butterfly or small-caliber IV catheter. Common sites of placement of the catheter in pediatric patients include outer thighs, upper arms, and abdomen (avoiding the area covered by a diaper). Intermittent dosing or continuous infusions can be used with subcutaneous catheters with a maximum infusion rate of 2 or 3 ml/hr depending on the catheter type. The catheter may need to be changed every 7–10 days or sooner if redness or swelling is noticed at insertion site. Rotation of location of insertion may prevent breakdown of skin in the area of the catheter. Careful selection of medications should occur prior to being given to ensure compatibility of medication to be given in the subcutaneous space. Some medications are caustic to subcutaneous tissues and should be avoided. Other medications commonly used in palliative care, such as lorazepam, burn when administered subcutaneously and should also be avoided.

TRANSDERMAL

Transdermal delivery of medications can include patches, creams, and gels, although the evidence for efficacy of compounded pain creams and gels is lacking. The most common pain medication given transdermally is a fentanyl patch. Fentanyl patches can be a useful way to give sustained opioids to pediatric patients without them needing to swallow a pill of an extended-release opioid. Fentanyl dosing can be a barrier to usage because the smallest dose patch available is the 12 μg/hr patch, and the patch cannot be cut or covered by an occlusive film. In infants and small children, the smallest fentanyl dose patch may exceed the daily oral morphine equivalent intake to be safely used. In children with illnesses affecting skin integrity such as epidermolysis bullosa, patches should be avoided because they should not be placed over broken skin or rashes.

INTRANASAL

Intranasal administration of medications has increased in recent years with the wider availability of atomizer devices. Many medications have been shown to be readily absorbed in the nasal mucosa and can be reliably dosed in pediatric patients. Utilizing intranasal opioids can be a way to avoid the gastrointestinal track, painful injections, and risks to intravenous access. Intranasal medications can yield quick onset of action, good bioavailability, avoid first-pass metabolism, and have good tolerability among pediatric patients. Changes in mucosa and ciliary clearance may affect drug uptake, especially in patients with large cleft palate defects and cystic fibrosis or ciliopathy. Evidence is building on the many uses of the intranasal route for palliative symptom management, including respiratory distress, intermittent pain, palliative births, and sedations. No large randomized controlled trials have been performed; however, to date, the best evidence of efficacy exists for intranasal fentanyl, ketamine, midazolam, and dexmedetomidine.

INHALED

Inhaled medication delivery has been used for decades; however, there is limited evidence supporting its use in pain management of palliative patients. Smaller trials have shown benefit of inhaled morphine and fentanyl in patients with end-stage lung disease experiencing breathlessness. They may have a role for pediatric patients with the inability to tolerate other routes of delivery. Inhaled opioids avoid first-pass metabolism; however, patients may still experience some of the side effects of systemic absorption such as constipation and sedation. Morphine and hydromorphone may trigger a release of histamine and may worsen bronchoconstriction in patients predisposed to airway reactivity, so some providers choose inhaled fentanyl instead. Inhaled medication delivery is usually well tolerated in pediatric patients at many developmental stages. However, this modality is not as easily transported, and the patient may need a different route of medication during travel outside the home.

RECTAL

The rectal route of drug delivery has been used for centuries, especially at end of life when patients are no longer able to take oral medications or have gastrointestinal dysfunction. Rectally administered medications are easy to use, and family members can be taught how to administer them. Most oral medications can be given per rectum (PR) with the same dosing guidelines. Suppositories are commercially available for some medications; however, many medications can be compounded into suppositories or the pill or liquid suspension given PR. Some pediatric patients, especially adolescents and young adults, may not tolerate medications given PR due to privacy concerns, and these topics should be explored prior to administration of medications PR. Rectal administration should be avoided in patients with neutropenia, thrombocytopenia, and those with rectal disease.

SUMMARY

Returning to the case example, the neonate with gastroschisis with agitation and pain was finally comfortable with IV fentanyl but now has no IV or enteral access. It would be reasonable to develop a short-term plan for today and to plan for longer term access. To ensure the neonate's immediate comfort, you can add intranasal fentanyl for intermittent dosing. You may need to coordinate with your pharmacy for dosing and for the atomizer intranasal delivery device. A long-term plan for this neonate should include IV access, but there might be a delay in getting long-term access such as a PICC line or other central line placed. If the neonate needs a continuous infusion of opioid, you can place a subcutaneous catheter and start the fentanyl infusion through this access route. The subcutaneous catheter can give you days to arrange for a long-term access route and still maintain adequate analgesia.

Selecting the appropriate route of pain medication should be individualized based on pain type, severity, prognosis, and developmental age of the pediatric patient. Discussing options with caregivers and exploring the benefits and burdens of each route of medication delivery can help determine the most effective and least distressing route.

KEY POINTS TO REMEMBER

- Use the least invasive route first.
- Match route with developmental level and neurologic capability of child.
- Explore benefits and burdens of potential routes with patient and caregiver.
- Remember there are medication delivery routes other than oral and IV that may be beneficial to pediatric patients.

Further Reading

Beckwith, C, Feddema, SS, Barton, RG, Graves C. A guide to drug therapy in patients with enteral feeding tubes: Dosage form selection and administration methods. *Hosp Pharm.* 2004;39(3):225–237.

Harlos MS, Stenekes S, Lambert D, Hohl C, Chochinov HM. Intranasal fentanyl in the palliative care of newborns and infants. *J Pain Symptom Manage.* 2013;46(2):265–274.

Patel A, Jacobsen L, Jhaveri R, Bradford KK. Effectiveness of pediatric pill swallowing interventions: A systematic review. *Pediatrics.* 2015;135(5):883–889.

Pieper L, Wager J, Zernikow B. Intranasal fentanyl for respiratory distress in children and adolescents with life-limiting conditions. *BMC Palliat Care.* 2018;17(1):106.

17 My Skin Feels Like It Is on Fire

Lindsay B. Ragsdale

You are asked to see a 14-year-old male with an unknown rheumatologic disease who presented with intense burning and swelling in his left lower extremity. His pain has intensified in the past week, affecting his ability to ambulate and resulting in sleep disruption. His lower leg and foot are swollen and erythematous with scattered papules. He has pain with light brushing of the top of his foot and cannot tolerate an exam of his leg. His pain has affected his mood, and he has withdrawn from his friends and activities. He is also scheduled for a biopsy of the skin on his leg tomorrow, and he is scared about the pain this biopsy will cause him. He is tearful and rates his burning pain a 9/10 and constant. He describes his pain as feeling like his skin is on fire. He asks you to help him with his pain and to create a strategy to get him through his biopsy tomorrow.

What do you do now?

NEUROPATHIC PAIN

Neuropathic pain is the painful sensation arising from direct damage or a disease affecting the somatosensory system. Although the exact mechanisms are unknown, emerging theories indicate that neuropathic pain could be more complex than just direct damage or disease; it could involve dysfunction in pain processing centers. There is limited evidence about the assessment and treatment of neuropathic pain in pediatrics. There are some challenges to assessing and managing neuropathic pain due to developmental age, expressive language ability, no validated neuropathic assessment tools in children, and a paucity of medications approved for this indication for pediatrics (Table 17.1). However, emerging evidence and expert opinion have shed some light on a stepwise, multimodal approach to this type of pain.

Assessment of pain in children should be matched to their developmental level and capability to gain the most accurate depiction. Many validated somatic pain assessments in pediatrics exist; the most commonly used are the Faces, Legs, Activity, Cry, and Consolability (FLACC), numerical rating, and Wong–Baker FACES® scales. Pain history should include location, intensity, timing, quality, and alleviating and aggravating factors. However, to capture the nature of neuropathic pain, further exploration of neuropathic

TABLE 17.1 **Treatments for Neuropathic Pain**

Treatment	Medication
First line	Gabapentin/pregabalin
	Duloxetine
	Amitriptyline
Second line	Clonidine
	Ketamine
	Topical lidocaine
Refractory	Opioids including methadone
	Interventional modalities
Adjunct	Integrative therapies

sensations is needed beyond a standard pain history. You must ask the patient about sensations of prickling, tingling, pins and needles, shock or shooting, hot or burning, numbness, flushing, and excessive sweating in the affected area. Although these concepts are difficult for infants and younger children or ones with developmental delay, some children can conceptualize sensations and are able to describe them in their own words. They may be able to describe pain based on concrete experiences they have had before in their life, such as pins and needles sensation after sitting in one place too long or burning sensation. Hyperalgesia is pain out of proportion to a minimally painful stimulus. Allodynia is extreme pain with non-noxious touch, such as 10/10 pain with a bedsheet touching the affected area. Both of these types of sensory responses are reflective of neuropathic-type pain impulses and should also be assessed during history and physical exam. Assessing for these more difficult sensations may require patience and creativity for the clinician.

Once neuropathic pain has been diagnosed, treatment strategy should depend on pain timing and intensity. Some postoperative neuropathic pain may be milder and short-lived and may not require systemic therapy. However, some neuropathic pain can be chronic and debilitating, and without treatment it can significantly affect the patient's and the family's quality of life. Meticulous symptom management for patients with chronic neuropathic pain can help prevent effects on mood, activity level, and functionality. A multimodal approach will likely give the best results, but the treatment strategy should be tailored to each pediatric patient.

Integrative therapies such as diaphragmatic breathing, biofeedback, guided imagery, aromatherapy, acupuncture, and expressive arts can be a useful adjunct to a pain strategy. Finding ways to harness children's connection with their bodies and give them tools to help find control over some aspect of their pain can empower the children and reduce feelings of helplessness. Although robust research is lacking on many integrative therapies in children, layering in these supports into a medication regimen may be of benefit and can potentially improve pain scores in some children.

To date, few randomized controlled trials have been performed on systemic medications to treat neuropathic pain in children, and the evidence for their effectiveness is weak. Current evidence supports gabapentinoids (gabapentin/pregabalin) and antidepressants (duloxetine and amitriptyline) as first-line treatment of neuropathic pain in pediatrics. Gabapentin is the most common initial neuropathic agent and can be well tolerated in children. The most common side effects are sedation and dizziness. Efficacy may be seen within a few days, or titration may be needed for maximal benefit. Titration of the dose should occur every few days to prevent excessive sedation, with the goal of finding the lowest therapeutic dose. Some patients may respond to pregabalin that failed gabapentin, and a rotation may be beneficial. Some challenges may exist with insurers not approving pregabalin unless there is documented failure of gabapentin beforehand.

Serotonin–norepinephrine reuptake inhibitor (SNRI) antidepressants such as duloxetine and venlafaxine have been shown to be beneficial in the treatment of neuropathic pain in pediatrics. Duloxetine has more evidence to support its use in neuropathic pain and can be particularly helpful in patients with overlying mood disturbances such as depression or anxiety. Amitriptyline is a tricyclic antidepressant (TCA) that has also shown efficacy in neuropathic pain in pediatrics. Efficacy with these agents may not be seen for several weeks, and this may warrant a strategy to manage the pain during this titration period. Due to their sedative effect, TCAs can be particularly helpful in patients with sleep disruption. Monitoring for side effects such as nausea, sexual dysfunction, and suicidal ideations is important, especially during the initiation period. TCAs have a potential overdose risk when prescribed for home use, and caution should be used with patients with a history of depression and suicidality.

Emerging evidence suggests that low-dose methadone and ketamine are potentially beneficial agents for neuropathic pain. Methadone is a μ-opioid receptor agonist and N-methyl-D-aspartate (NMDA) antagonist; the latter action makes it a potential neuropathic agent. Methadone can be difficult to dose in pediatrics; however, in refractory cases of neuropathic pain, it may be a helpful treatment. The liquid formulation makes it more convenient for dosing for smaller children and infants, and it may also be administered via enteral feeding tube. Ketamine also has effects on NMDA receptors and can relieve neuropathic pain at subanesthetic dosing. Ketamine can be administered intravenously (IV) or intranasally, and the IV solution can be taken by mouth. Side effects of ketamine include dissociative mental status, hallucinations, nystagmus, increased intracranial pressure, and increased secretion production. Availability of ketamine in the community, abuse and diversion potential, and insurance approval may be challenges to its routine use.

Opioids (e.g., morphine, hydromorphone, and fentanyl) are not recommended as first-line treatment for neuropathic pain and should be used only in cases of refractory pain despite using multiple other agents. Some pediatric patients have such severe pain, especially at end of life, that using strong opioids may be the only way to ease their suffering. Discussing risks and burdens of strong opioids with the patient and family can set expectations for pain control and potential side effects such as sedation, constipation, and nausea.

Topical agents may have a role in neuropathic pain management, especially peripheral neuropathy isolated to a small area. There is evidence that lidocaine patches and capsaicin patches provide temporary relief of neuropathic pain localized to discrete areas. Lidocaine patches can be used daily and can be cut to fit any shape. Side effects can include erythema of the patch site, but overall they are well tolerated with little systemic absorption. Some over-the-counter lidocaine patches are available and may be easy for patients to trial. Capsaicin 8% patches have stronger evidence in the adult literature for diabetic neuropathy, but this etiology of neuropathic pain is rare in pediatrics. Capsaicin patches can be placed in the area for 30–60 minutes every few months with sustained downregulation of receptor activity in the area. Pediatric data for capsaicin usage are not currently available, but capsaicin may be an option in refractory cases in adolescents and young adult patients. Capsaicin cream can be particularly painful to use at first, especially at high doses, so anticipatory guidance should be given to patients who choose to try this modality.

Interventional modalities can have a role in refractory neuropathic pain in pediatrics. Regional pain blocks and nerve catheter placements can help control isolated neuropathic pain. The underlying etiology and prognosis should be considered with regional nerve blocks and catheters because they are not always a long-term solution, but they can help with refractory pain in palliative patients with days to weeks or even months prognosis. If the expertise in pediatric interventional pain is available, nerve ablation techniques can be pursued for patients with a longer expected survival because they can give long-term pain relief for some patients.

Our case of the 14-year-old boy with burning neuropathic pain of his left leg requires a multimodal approach to his pain regimen. You should first take a thorough pain history, paying close attention to the pain intensity, timing, and modulating factors. Your exam should closely evaluate his leg, paying attention to his reaction to palpation, light touch, and movement. After establishing his pain is due to neuropathic pain, you start him on gabapentin three times a day with a plan to titrate up in 3 days. You discuss his biopsy plan with his rheumatologist, who agrees to involve pediatric anesthesiology prior to the biopsy. The anesthesiologist performs a regional block of his leg prior to biopsy and will monitor the potential need for a sustained nerve block with the placement of a nerve catheter. You integrate child life into his pain plan with attention to preoperative readiness and relaxation techniques. After you describe the plan to him, he takes a deep breath and relaxes in bed feeling relieved that someone is going to control his pain. His biopsy occurs without issues, and his nerve block controls his pain during the procedure. His neuropathic pain improves during the next few days as he awaits the biopsy results. He starts to smile more throughout the next few days and is more engaged in activities that make him happy.

KEY POINTS TO REMEMBER

- Perform detailed pain history and exam with attention to neuropathic sensations.
- First-line therapy is gabapentin/pregabalin, SNRIs, and TCAs.
- Integrative therapies are useful as adjunct to pharmacologic therapies.

Further Reading

Madden K, Bruera E. Very-low-dose methadone to treat refractory neuropathic pain in children with cancer. *J Palliat Med.* 2017;20(11):1280–1283.

Sommer C, Cruccu G. Topical treatment of peripheral neuropathic pain: Applying the evidence. *J Pain Symptom Manage.* 2017;53(3):614–629.

Windsor RB, Tham SW, Adams TL, Anderson A. The use of opioids for the treatment of pediatric neuropathic pain. *Clin J Pain.* 2019;35:509–514.

18 The Withdrawn Child

Ricki Carroll and Carly Levy

You are consulted on a 14-year-old female with spastic quadriplegic cerebral palsy, intellectual disability, generalized epilepsy, gastroesophageal reflux, and bowel dysmotility. Her mother brought her to the emergency department due to change in behavior. Her mother reports her daughter has been shrieking, sweating, and "just not acting herself" for days. Her mother states that her daughter has been having similar episodes for the past 6 months, but they usually resolve. Her pediatrician had obtained labs, and she had a neurology follow-up appointment in which an electroencephalogram (EEG) was performed. She has been admitted for further workup. On exam, she is lying in bed moaning and grimacing. She does not make eye contact but instead keeps her gaze fixed on the ceiling. Her heart rate is 102 beats per minute, and her blood pressure is 134/75 mmHg. Her exam is notable for frequent myoclonus of her extremities. Her mother is at her bedside visibly upset and insistent that something is wrong.

What do you do now?

PAIN IN THE NEUROLOGICALLY IMPAIRED CHILD

The assessment of pain in children with neurologic impairment can be challenging. In addition to not being able to articulate distress, neurologically impaired children may not recognize the sensation as pain or may experience it in a different way. They may express their distress through a range of ritualized pain behaviors, such as vocalizations, facial expressions, or restlessness. Some children may have more atypical behaviors, such as laughter, withdrawal, or listlessness. It can be difficult to differentiate these actions from other nonverbal cues, creating additional barriers to recognizing pain, detecting patterns, and identifying potential pain sources. Implementing an individualized pain assessment tool, focused on pain behaviors in nonverbal children, can be helpful to both parents and providers as a way to document signs of discomfort specific to that child and to assess and monitor pain over time.

Pain is a significant problem for children with neurologic impairment. Studies have indicated that pain occurs more frequently and at a higher intensity in these children than the average population. There are various reasons for this (Table 18.1). One contributing factor is that children with neurologic impairment are at greater risk for certain problems that are uncommon in childhood and can cause acute, chronic, and/or recurrent pain. This can be due to exposure to certain medications, such as antiepileptic medications that can cause gallstones and pancreatitis, or due to specialized formulas or diets, such as a ketogenic diet that can increase risk for kidney stones and urinary tract infections. The source of pain can also be due to a symptom inherent in central nervous system (CNS) impairment, such as hypertonicity leading to hip subluxation or the inability to ambulate leading to osteoporosis and increased risk for fracture.

In addition to these uncommon sources of nociceptive pain in childhood, it is important to bear in mind that children with neurologic impairment can experience common childhood causes of discomfort as well, such as gastroesophageal reflux (GERD) and urinary tract infections. Furthermore, individuals with injury to the CNS may have impairment in the balance between inhibition and excitation nerve signals. This imbalance in signals can also lead to improper or heightened firing of pain fibers, leading to central neuropathic pain or visceral hyperalgesia. As a result, even common sources of pain in childhood can be amplified in intensity or in frequency when experienced by a child with neurologic impairment.

TABLE 18.1 Sources of Pain in Children with Neurologic Impairment

Common Childhood Sources That Can Be Amplified	Rare Childhood Sources That Are More Common	Sources Due to Central Nervous System Impairment	Iatrogenic Causes
Teething	Dental decay	Hypertonicity/spasticity/ contractures	Medication side effects/toxicity profile
Otitis media	Gallstones	Myoclonus	
Gastroesophageal reflux	Pancreatitis	Dystonia	Medication withdrawal
Constipation	Bladder distention	Dysautonomia	
Urinary tract infection	Hip subluxation	Neuropathic pain (central or peripheral)	
Fracture	Pressure sores	Visceral hyperalgesia	
	Self-inflicted injuries		

Another possible contributing factor is symptoms intrinsic to neurologic dysfunction. Following CNS injury, it is common for individuals to suffer from a variety of symptoms related to the injury, including myoclonus, dystonia, and autonomic dysfunction, depending on the location and type of injury. Symptoms range from intermittent muscle spasms to prolonged episodes of flushing, tachycardia, hypertension, hyperthermia, and diaphoresis. These symptoms may be present rarely or on a daily basis, and they may or may not cause discomfort, but they are likely to escalate during episodes of heightened emotion, such as pain, anxiety, or agitation. In other words, these symptoms may be a primary source of discomfort, or pain from another source can induce or increase these features, creating a secondary source of pain.

Providers should also consider iatrogenic causes. Commonly, children with neurologic impairment have associated comorbidities, leading to an array of medical specialists, multiple daily medications, and frequent medication adjustments. Many medications have side effects, toxicity profiles, and/or can cause withdrawal symptoms that are similar to pain behaviors.

For your patient, it is clear that her current behaviors are indicating to her mother a change in her baseline that is suggestive of her being in pain. It is also evident that although she is experiencing an acute episode of pain, she has been suffering from episodic pain for quite some time. A workup has already been initiated in the outpatient setting. The next steps will include obtaining (1) an in-depth history, including historical and current medications; (2) a thorough physical exam; (3) the results of the outpatient lab work and EEG; and then (4) any additional diagnostic tests to identify the source of the pain, using Table 18.1 as a guide.

Her outpatient lab work and EEG as well as inpatient labs and urine samples are found to be unremarkable. On further discussion with her mother, some of her pain episodes seem to subside following a bowel movement. A detailed history reveals that she has a significant history of constipation and is on a bowel regimen including a stool softener and a motility agent. In the past, she stooled every day, but since starting her menses earlier this year, she has been stooling less frequently. You recommend an abdominal X-ray, which confirms significant stool burden, and she is administered an enema with good result. She is back to her baseline overnight but has a recurrence of her pain episode the following day.

For many children such as the child described in this chapter, no source is identified or the child continues to display pain behaviors despite treatment of a possible source. Although it is important to consider further studies, this is also the time to consider empiric treatment trials that target pain related to CNS impairment (Figure 18.1). The best studied medications for these pain sources are gabapentin, pregabalin, and tricyclic antidepressants. Other medications to consider include serotonin–norepinephrine reuptake inhibitors, antiepileptic medications, antispasmodic medications, α_2 agonists, N-methyl-D-aspartic acid receptor antagonists, opioids, and cannabinoids. Scheduled acetaminophen or as-needed ibuprofen may be beneficial. In addition, empirical treatment of GERD is often initiated or optimized at this time or earlier because this is a common and important source of pain to consider in children with neurologic impairment. If there is suspicion that pain could be related to gastric dysmotility and constipation, a bowel regimen should be initiated or maximized, which may include daily gentle suppositories or enemas.

When embarking on an empirical approach, there are some important considerations to take into account. First, be sure to define criteria for starting and stopping medications; these are time-limited trials and will require frequent reassessment. Set up reasonable expectations, including that this can be a lengthy process and that it may not completely resolve the symptoms. Use a systematic approach, trialing as few medications and making as few changes as possible at a time. Finally, many children with neurologic impairment and persistent pain behaviors benefit from a combination of nonpharmacologic interventions and a medication trial. Comfort strategies include cuddling/swaddling, rocking, massaging, warm baths, and pleasurable activities such as listening to music. Environmental modifications could include changes in temperature, light, or sound. Equipment to consider includes supportive pillows for positional pain, weighted blankets, and vibrating mats and pillows for vibratory stimulation. For gastrointestinal-related distress in children with a feeding tube, strategies include venting the gastrostomy tube and decreasing the volume and/or rate of fluids. Integrative therapies, such as aromatherapy, acupuncture, and biofeedback, may also be beneficial for certain children.

The child in our case is likely experiencing pain and cramping due to constipation. However, she may also be experiencing visceral hyperalgesia related to her intestinal distention. In addition, her pain episodes, which

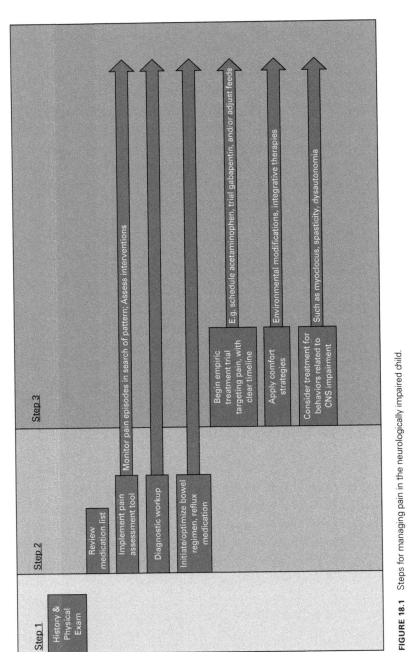

FIGURE 18.1 Steps for managing pain in the neurologically impaired child.

include flushing, sweating, and sustained myoclonus, are distressing for her and her mother. Her treatment plan should include not only a stepwise bowel regimen but also interventions focused on her distressing symptoms. It may be advantageous to initiate a neuropathic agent to treat hyperalgesia or to trial an as-needed α agonist at the start of a pain episode. Certainly, the other key component to her treatment plan should focus on nonpharmacologic strategies that may help augment a medication trial.

KEY POINTS TO REMEMBER

- The first step in assessing a neurologically impaired child with pain behaviors is conducting an in-depth history and physical exam.
- Pain is a significant problem for children with neurologic impairment. This specific population has additional sources of nociceptive and neuropathic pain that must be considered.
- When tailoring a treatment plan, consider therapeutic interventions for the presumed etiology as well as for the associated pain and symptoms.
- An empirical approach is reasonable when the etiology remains unclear; ensure a systematic method, and define criteria for starting and stopping medications when first initiating. Set up reasonable expectations, and provide families with anticipatory guidance about possible outcomes with starting time-limited trials.
- Nonpharmacologic interventions are always an important part of symptom management.

Further Reading

Hadden KL, von Baeyer CL. Pain in children with cerebral palsy: Common triggers and expressive behaviors. *Pain.* 2002;99(1–2):281–288.

Hauer JM. *Caring for Children Who Have Severe Neurologic Impairment.* Baltimore, MD: Johns Hopkins University Press; 2013.

Houlihan C, O'Donnell M, Conaway M, Stevenson R. Bodily pain and health-related quality of life in children with cerebral palsy. *Dev Med Child Neurol.* 2004;46(5):305–310.

19 She Won't Stop Vomiting

Carly Levy and Mindy Dickerman

A consult is requested for a 12-year-old girl with acute myeloid leukemia (AML) who was readmitted yesterday for a round of chemotherapy. The medical team is seeking advice to help relieve her intractable nausea and vomiting that started on admission. Upon further questioning, she has a history of poorly controlled chemotherapy-induced nausea and vomiting for which she was treated with various combinations of ondansetron, diphenhydramine, granisetron, aprepitant, and dexamethasone with limited success. She describes this episode of nausea and vomiting as different than previous episodes. She notes her nausea preceded the initiation of chemotherapy. She reports stooling regularly and denies any other associated symptoms—no fever, diarrhea, or abdominal pain. Her nausea is not triggered by specific foods or odors, and no new medications have been started recently. The team started scheduled ondansetron and diphenhydramine without relief.

What do you do now?

NAUSEA AND VOMITING

Nausea and vomiting can be a significant source of suffering for patients with advanced illness. Several studies reveal nausea and vomiting occur in almost half of children with cancer during their end-of-life period. While attempting to determine the etiology for the patient's symptoms, it is important to keep in mind goals of care when tailoring the appropriate therapeutic interventions. Decisions about location of management (inpatient vs. outpatient) as well as the level of aggressiveness (medical ± surgical) will be based on both degree of suffering and the patient's/family's goals of care. Management should include combining pharmacology with supportive and integrative therapies.

PATHOPHYSIOLOGY

When evaluating a patient with advanced illness who is suffering from nausea and vomiting, providers should have an appreciation of the complex neurophysiology responsible for these symptoms (Figure 19.1). The vomiting reflex is activated by a group of neurons in the medulla known as the vomiting center. The vomiting center receives feedback directly from four sources: the gastrointestinal tract, the chemoreceptor trigger zone, the cerebral cortex, and the vestibular apparatus in the inner ear. Specific neurotransmitters stimulate the vomiting center; consequently, therapeutic interference with these neurotransmitters can mitigate activation. Therapies should be initiated based on the presumed mechanism of nausea and the transmitters that are implicated.

The chemoreceptor trigger zone is located in the area postrema, which is located on the floor of the fourth ventricle. It responds to the accumulation of toxins in the blood and/or cerebrospinal fluid from either medication (i.e., antibiotics, opioids, corticosteroids, nonsteroidal inflammatory drugs, anticholinergics, and chemotherapeutic agents) or a metabolic disturbance (uremia from renal failure, hypercalcemia, hyponatremia, ketoacidosis, etc.). The primary neurotransmitters involved in this pathway include serotonin ($5\text{-}HT_3$) and dopamine (D_2). In contrast, the cerebral cortex responds to increasing intracranial pressure and/or conditioned responses, including memories or experiences associated with emotional distress, primarily fear and anxiety.

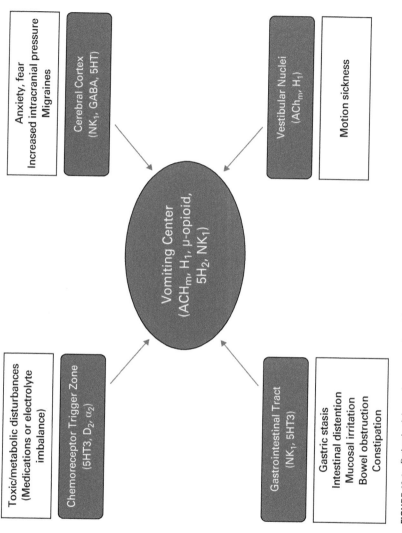

FIGURE 19.1 Pathophysiology of nausea and vomiting.

The gastrointestinal system is a common stimulus leading to activation of the vomiting center. Substances such as acids, local tissue damage, and mechanical forces in the gastrointestinal tract can stimulate nausea and vomiting. Local irritation of the gastrointestinal tract can be triggered by common medications such as nonsteroidal anti-inflammatory drugs or antibiotics. Local gastrointestinal tissue damage can be caused by tumor, radiation, or infection. Distention of the gastrointestinal tract from constipation, obstruction, or even tube feedings are additional causes of nausea. Nausea due to intestinal obstruction is thought to be associated with an inflammatory response causing release of prostaglandins, secretagogues, and nocioceptive mediators. Finally, swallowed blood or secretions and the gag reflex can stimulate nausea and vomiting.

CLINICAL APPROACH

In general, the approach to these patients should include a thorough history and physical examination to identify the possible etiology while confirming goals of care before developing the plan (Figure 19.2). Providers should ask about the nature of the vomiting—whether it is bilious, projectile, or bloody. In addition, it is important to note the pattern or timing of the symptoms to determine if they are associated with any particular triggers, including odors, meals, or medications. Associated symptoms should be solicited (i.e., fever, diarrhea, pain, headaches, constipation, heartburn, or emotional distress). Younger patients may have difficulty distinguishing between pain and nausea. A careful review of the patient's medication history should be conducted. On physical exam, pay close attention to the abdominal and neurologic exam. Localized tenderness may lead a provider to consider a gastrointestinal source, whereas focal neurologic findings including positional pain, papilledema, and changes in vision, speech, coordination, or gait may steer one to consider an underlying intracranial process.

When attempting to determine the etiology, measures should be taken to avoid certain odors while offering small, frequent, desirable meals. Providers should implement age-appropriate cognitive–behavioral strategies such as relaxation exercises, controlled breathing, and guided imagery. Younger children may require facilitation, whereas older children can be taught self-hypnosis. Unlike pharmacologic treatments for nausea, hypnosis has few,

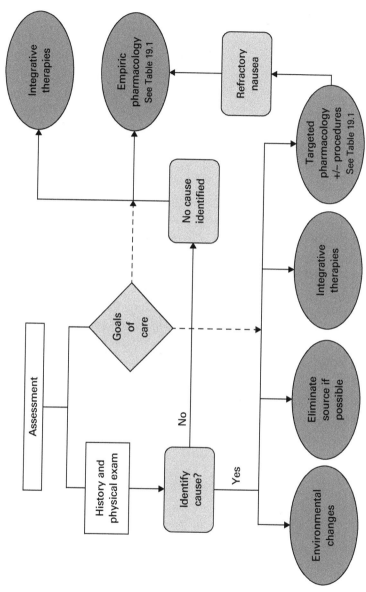

FIGURE 19.2 Stepwise approach to nausea and vomiting.

if any, side effects and can facilitate a sense of control in children with advanced illness. If the etiology is identified, steps should be taken to reverse or reduce the stimulus, as long as the interventions remain in line with the patient's goals of care.

When symptoms are due to stimulation of the chemoreceptor trigger zone (i.e., medications or metabolic disturbances), providers should first consider discontinuing or rotating medication(s) and/or correcting of electrolyte abnormalities, when feasible. For refractory symptoms, select medications that target the blockade of neurotransmitters involved in this pathway, primarily serotonin and dopamine (Table 19.1).

Similarly, the approach to symptoms stemming from the stimulation of the cerebral cortex should also address the underlying cause (see Table 19.1). When treating patients with symptoms secondary to central nervous system tumors or metastatic disease, the first-line agent should address increased intracranial pressure (i.e., dexamethasone). On the other hand, patients with severe anticipatory nausea, akin to the patient described in the case in this chapter, might respond well to integrative and supportive modalities, in addition to an anxiolytic medication (i.e., lorazepam).

If the patient's history and physical exam determine the cause of nausea to be from the gastrointestinal tract, therapy can be targeted to treat the specific source (see Table 19.1). Constipation should be treated aggressively with diet and medications. Medications that may be causing gastric irritation or constipation should be evaluated for their continued benefit and alternatives considered. Antacid therapy can be initiated when gastritis is suspected. Prokinetic agents, such as metoclopramide, may help with gastric stasis or intestinal dysmotility. Children with severe neurologic impairment suspected of having visceral hyperalgesia can receive an empiric trial of gabapentin.

Providers should maintain a high index of suspicion for bowel obstruction in children with advanced cancer or a history of abdominal surgeries. The primary goal when treating these patients should be to alleviate pain and nausea while allowing oral intake, if still desired. Treatment recommendations should be guided by the location of obstruction and the patient's prognosis, functional status, and goals of care. Options may include bowel resection; placement of a venting gastrostomy tube; stent placement; or, for patients who opt for less invasive measures, medical management

TABLE 19.1   Pathways, Associated Causes, and Treatment of Nausea and Vomiting

Pathway/Cause	Treatment
Chemoreceptor trigger zone (5-HT$_3$, D$_2$, and α_2)	
Medications	Decrease, discontinue, or rotate medications if possible. 5-HT$_3$ antagonist (ondansetron or granisetron) D$_2$ antagonist (metoclopramide or haloperidol)
Metabolic disturbances	Correct disturbances.
Cerebral cortex (NK$_1$, GABA, and 5-HT)	
Central nervous system tumor	Corticosteroids (dexamethasone) Consider radiation therapy.
Conditioned response (anxiety, fear)	Counseling Integrative therapies Benzodiazepines
Gastrointestinal tract (NK$_1$ and 5-HT$_3$)	
Gastric irritation	Stop irritant. H$_2$ blocker or PPI
Constipation	Stool softener (docusate) Osmotic agents (polyethylene glycol and lactulose) Stimulant (senna) Enema
Tube feedings	Reduce or discontinue feedings.
Thick secretions	Nebulized saline expectorant
Bowel obstruction	Limit intake and consider nasogastric tube. Consider surgical options. Partial small bowel obstruction- metoclopramide Opioid + corticosteroid ± H$_2$ blocker/PPI Consider D$_2$ antagonist, anticholinergic, or octreotide.

(continued)

Table 10.1 **Continued**	
Pathway/Cause	Treatment
Refractory symptoms or unclear cause	
	First line
	5-HT$_3$ antagonist (ondansetron)
	Integrative strategies
	Second line (consider rotating to or adding)
	D$_2$ antagonist (olanzapine and haloperidol)
	Benzodiazepine
	Dexamethasone or diphenhydramine
	Third line
	Aprepitant
	Cannabinoids (dronabinol and medical marijuana)
	Low-dose propofol

PPI, proton pump inhibitor; 5-HT$_3$, 5-Hydroxytryptamine^3 receptor; D$_2$, Dopamine receptor; GABA, Gamma-Aminobutyric Acid receptor; NK$_1$, Neuokinine 1 receptor; H$_2$, Histamine H$_2$ receptor.

directed at reducing gastrointestinal secretions, nausea/vomiting, and pain. Prokinetic agents may be beneficial in partial obstruction but may exacerbate crampy abdominal pain and are contraindicated in complete bowel obstruction. Acid-suppressing medications are often used. Opioids and dopamine antagonists (i.e., haloperidol and olanzapine) can help relieve pain and nausea. Antimuscarinic/anticholinergic medications (glycopyrrolate and scopolamine) can treat colicky pain. Corticosteroids are used to decrease the inflammation and edema in the intestine as well as to relieve nausea. Somatostatin analogs, such as octreotide, administered subcutaneously or intravenously, have been used safely and may decrease nausea and vomiting associated with intestinal obstruction. Combination therapies are thought to be superior to using a single agent, but further study is needed to determine which combinations are best.

Opioid-induced nausea/vomiting is common in advanced illness and end of life. Opioids stimulate the chemoreceptor trigger zone and the vestibular apparatus, and they also cause intestinal dysmotility and constipation. Under these circumstances, nausea/vomiting typically begin immediately following opioid initiation and/or a recent dose titration. This usually resolves within a few days. If the symptoms persist, consider an opioid rotation or a low-dose naloxone infusion to reduce the frequency and severity of nausea without antagonizing the analgesic effect. Patients with opioid-induced constipation due to decreased bowel motility should be started on a bowel stimulant (i.e., senna). For select patients who remain constipated despite maximized bowel regimen, a trial of methylnaltrexone may be helpful. Methylnaltexone, a peripheral µ-opioid receptor antagonist that has restricted ability to cross the blood–brain barrier, has been demonstrated in adults to have good effect at relieving opioid-induced constipation without affecting analgesia or precipitating opiate withdrawal. Otherwise, for patients on chronic opioids suffering from persistent nausea and/or vomiting, providers should consider causes unrelated to opioids.

Cannabinoid receptor agonists (i.e., dronabinol and Δ-9-tetrahydrocannabinol) are US Food and Drug Administration approved for chemotherapy-induced nausea and vomiting and may be considered for refractory symptoms. Side effects of cannabinoid receptor agonists include dizziness, dysphoria, hallucinations, and hypotension, although children are thought to be less sensitive to the psychotropic effects. Families of children with advanced illness are increasingly interested in using medical marijuana to relieve nausea and vomiting. Although medical marijuana is a potential therapy to consider for treatment of refractory nausea, it remains clinically controversial due to the lack of empiric evidence on efficacy and safety, and access is variable depending on where a patient lives. Clinicians should use caution in recommending it to pediatric patients with advanced illness.

Finally, when removal or reversal of the stimulus for nausea is less feasible or if the etiology remains unclear, providers should empirically implement a multimodal approach. Supportive and integrative strategies should be offered while initiating medications in a stepwise manner (see Table 19.1). Choose the route of administration for each medication that ensures maximal drug bioavailability and is in line with the patient's/family's goals of care. As additional antiemetics are being considered and combination therapies being used, providers should consider potential risks and drug interactions. To ensure the best ongoing treatment plan for an individual patient's nausea/vomiting, providers should routinely re-evaluate the patient's symptoms, prognosis, and goals of care.

The 12-year-old with AML we are consulting on is likely experiencing anticipatory nausea given that the timing of her symptoms preceded the initiation of emetogenic medications and a negative review of systems. In this case, we suspect her prior experiences of intractable chemotherapy-induced nausea and vomiting are triggering significant anxiety that manifests as nausea/vomiting. Under these circumstances, providers should encourage age-appropriate cognitive–behavioral strategies such as hypnosis, relaxation exercises, controlled breathing, and guided imagery and a trial of an anxiolytic medication, such as lorazepam.

KEY POINTS TO REMEMBER

- Try to identify the etiology of nausea/vomiting by thorough history and exam.
- Initiate environmental changes and age-appropriate integrative modalities.
- Consider goals of care in the context of treatment recommendations.
- Based on the etiology, identify the pathway responsible for the symptoms.
- When choosing a medication, target a receptor specific to the pathway identified.
- Choose a route of administration to ensure maximum drug bioavailability.
- If combining antiemetics, review potential drug interactions.
- If no etiology is identified, consider starting empiric pharmacologic therapy.

Further Reading

Ananth, P, Reed-Weston, A, Wolfe, J. Medical marijuana in pediatric oncology: A review of the evidence and implication for practice. *Pediatr Blood Cancer.* 2018;65:e26826.

Dupus LL, Boodhan, S, et al. Guideline for the prevention of acute nausea and vomiting due to antineoplastic medication in pediatric cancer patients. *Pediatr Blood Cancer.* 2013;60:1073–1082.

Friedrichsdorf SJ, Drake R, Webster MI. Gastrointestinal symptoms. In Wolfe J, Hinds P, Sourkes B, eds. *Textbook of Interdisciplinary Pediatric Palliative Care.* Philadelphia, PA: Elsevier; 2011:311–334.

Hardy JR, Glare P, Yates P, Mann KA. Palliation of nausea and vomiting. In Cherny NI, Fallon MT, Kaasa S, Portenoy RK, Currow DC, eds. *Oxford Textbook of Palliative Medicine.* 5th ed. Oxford, UK: Oxford University Press; 2015:661–674.

Hesketh, P. Chemotherapy-induced nausea and vomiting. *N Engl J Med.* 2008;358:2482–2494.

Hornby PJ. Central neurocircuitry associated with emesis. *Am J Med.* 2001;111(Suppl 8A):106S.

Jalmsell L, Kreicbergs U, Onelov E, et al. Symptoms affecting children with malignancies during the last month of life: A nationwide follow-up. *Pediatrics.* 2006;117(4):1314–1320.

Santucci G, Mack J. Common gastrointestinal symptoms in pediatric palliative care: Nausea, vomiting, constipation, cachexia. *Pediatr Clin N Am.* 2007;54:673–689.

Twycross R, Wilcock A, ed. *Hospice and Palliative Care Formulary USA.* 2nd ed. Nottingham, UK: palliativedrugs.com; 2009. Retrieved from https://www.palliativedrugs.com

Wolfe J, Grier HE, Klar N, et al. Symptoms and suffering at end of life in children with cancer. *N Engl J Med.* 2000;342(5):326–333.

20 Can't Catch My Breath

Juliana H. O'Brien

You are called to see a 15-year-old female with a history of acute myeloid leukemia status post bone marrow transplant who unfortunately developed bronchiolitis obliterans. She is admitted to the hospital for a recurrent pneumothorax and shortness of breath with increased oxygen requirement at home. She is typically on 2 L of oxygen via nasal cannula at home but is now requiring 15 L via non-rebreather. Her small pneumothorax self-resolves by her second day of admission. Despite this, she is short of breath when standing to transfer to bedside commode and has transient hypoxemic episodes with oxygen saturations in the low 80s. She feels anxious with exertion when she cannot catch her breath. She is not a candidate for lung transplant due to her recent history of malignancy. This is her second admission for pneumothorax in 2 months, and her functioning and exercise tolerance have decreased rapidly.

What do you do now?

DYSPNEA WITH CHRONIC OR END-STAGE DISEASE

Dyspnea is defined as the patient's subjective complaint of feeling short of breath, which may or may not be accompanied by objective exam findings. Dyspnea is common in patients with chronic and end-stage diseases and may be overlooked and undertreated. Untreated dyspnea can contribute to and worsen symptoms of fatigue, pain, anxiety, depression, nausea, and anorexia. Assessment of dyspnea in pediatrics is difficult because young children may not have the communication skills to describe their experience, and children with neurologic impairment may be nonverbal. Prevalence of dyspnea in children with complex chronic conditions ranges from 49% to 80% in the last month of life.

Dyspnea occurs when the physiologic demands or perceived demands for oxygenation and ventilation are unmet. A patient's blood oxygen saturation and lab work can indicate whether their physiologic demands are being met, but regardless, a patient may still have shortness of breath due to the increased workload of meeting their oxygen demands. The anxiety associated with breathlessness then creates a vicious cycle; the sense of panic causes an increased respiratory rate, thus increasing the already unmet demand. Then, for patients with chronic breathlessness who will often reduce their activity level, they will become deconditioned and subsequently experience even worse breathlessness with exertion. It is a cycle that can quickly become difficult to regain control.

Our patient's bronchiolitis obliterans is a progressive condition, but it is possible that she could have an underlying cause to her current respiratory insufficiency that is reversible, such as pneumonia, pneumothorax, viral upper respiratory infection, or anemia. When evaluating any patient with dyspnea, it is important to look for and treat any reversible causes. Table 20.1 lists potential causes of dyspnea, both acute and progressive, but it is not an exhaustive list of differential diagnoses. Table 20.2 outlines potential general treatment options for breathlessness. We apply a systems-based approach to examine potential causes of dyspnea and potential treatment options.

TABLE 20.1 Potential Causes of Dyspnea

Anatomic	Upper airway malformations or stenosis, malignancy—solid tumors compressing airways, and scoliosis
Neurologic	Central apnea and bulbar dysfunction
Cardiovascular	Anemia, congestive heart failure, pulmonary hypertension, and congenital heart disease
Respiratory	Parenchymal—asthma, pneumonia, and cystic fibrosis Extraparenchymal—pleural effusion, pneumothorax, and hemothorax
Gastrointestinal	Ascites and constipation
Musculoskeletal	Spinal muscular atrophy and muscular dystrophy

ANATOMIC

The inability to easily pull air into and out of the lungs due to obstruction or restriction may cause dyspnea. Infants with congenital facial or upper airway anomalies can experience dyspnea that may be responsive to noninvasive positive pressure ventilation or even better managed with a tracheostomy as a means to bypass their upper airway obstruction. Patients with neuromuscular scoliosis may have restricted lung capacity and thus develop dyspnea and chronic respiratory infections. Surgical scoliosis repair, if indicated, may improve their lung capacity and thus lessen or relieve dyspnea, but respiratory

TABLE 20.2 Treatments for Dyspnea

Evaluation and treatment of reversible causes
Upright positioning
Cool room temperature
Fan to the face
Pursed lip breathing
Self-hypnosis and guided imagery
Opioids
Benzodiazepines
Palliative sedation for severe end-of-life cases

issues in these children are often multifactorial. In cancer patients, if a solid tumor is compressing the airways causing dyspnea, treatment might include radiation, chemotherapy, and even surgical resection or debulking.

NEUROLOGIC

Patients with central apnea may experience significant distress related to dyspnea, and these patients may be verbal or nonverbal. For cognitively intact patients, it is extremely distressing to be aware of their need to breathe but be unable to do so. Unfortunately, children with severe neurologic impairment often suffer from central apnea but cannot verbalize their experience of dyspnea. These patients may need noninvasive positive airway pressure and, depending on the severity of central apnea, may need to consider a tracheostomy for chronic mechanical ventilation if it aligns with their goals of care.

For patients with bulbar dysfunction, advances in home airway clearance maneuvers with chest physiotherapy vests and mechanical insufflation–exsufflation machines and secretion management have helped these patients live longer and more comfortably. But despite these advancements, patients with progressive neuromuscular disease and subsequent severe bulbar dysfunction will eventually be faced with the decision about goals related to advanced technology, including options for tracheostomy for airway protection, airway clearance, and disease-directed management of their dyspnea.

Children with severe neurologic impairment may suffer a variety of respiratory problems, including weak cough, aspiration, hypoventilation due to muscle weakness, recurrent pneumonias, mucus plugging, and restrictive lung disease due to neuromuscular scoliosis. Disease-directed treatments including airway clearance techniques, noninvasive positive pressure ventilation, anticholinergics/botox/salivary duct ligation for oral secretion management, gastrostomy tubes with a fundoplication to avoid aspiration, and posterior spinal fusion have all shown some improvement in symptom control in this population. However, there is a risk that dyspnea persists in these children despite all of the disease-mitigating and life-prolonging treatments. Prior to any major treatment decision, providers should engage in goals-of-care conversations with caregivers to weigh the benefits and burdens of treatment.

CARDIOVASCULAR

Patients with shortness of breath secondary to end-stage congestive heart failure may respond to diuretics and oxygen. If the patient's dyspnea is distressing, you could consider concurrent use of opioids and benzodiazepines for symptom relief. Patients with end-stage congenital heart disease may also develop recurrent pleural effusions nearing the end of life. Prior to draining a pleural effusion, you must carefully consider the risk of circulatory collapse for these fragile patients and also consider managing their effusions conservatively with fluid restriction and diuretics.

RESPIRATORY

Examples of parenchymal sources of dyspnea include pneumonia, cystic fibrosis, and asthma. You should attempt to treat the primary source first if the treatment required is in line with the patient's goals of care. Treatment with antibiotics, inhaled bronchodilators, inhaled steroids, mucolytics, and systemic steroids can be utilized as appropriate. Patients who already have a daily regimen of airway clearance maneuvers may need to increase the frequency of their airway clearance during times of increased dyspnea.

Extraparenchymal causes of dyspnea can include pleural effusion, pneumothorax, hemothorax, and intrathoracic tumors that lead to atelectasis. Malignant pleural effusions can be seen in end-stage cancer, but depending on the individual's cancer and goals of care, the malignant pleural effusion may be a problem for months prior to death. Palliative options for malignant pleural effusions include serial thoracentesis, pleuradesis, or a long-term pleural catheter that can be intermittently drained at home. Shortness of breath caused by intrathoracic tumors may be alleviated with radiation, chemotherapy, and/or surgical resection. However, these patients may still benefit from opioids and benzodiazepines for symptom relief while receiving or awaiting tumor-directed treatment.

GASTROINTESTINAL

Ascites is a common cause of shortness of breath at the end of life due to abdominal competition on the diaphragm. A cancer patient who develops malignant ascites due to peritoneal carcinomatosis or liver metastasis has a very poor prognosis, often dying within weeks to months. Symptomatic relief may be achieved with either serial paracentesis or long-term peritoneal drain placement for home use. Malignant ascites can be very painful. Patients should be treated with opioids and benzodiazepines as needed concurrently with periodic drainage.

Ascites is also seen in patients with end-stage liver disease and portal hypertension. In pediatric patients, this might be seen not only in those with a primary liver diagnosis but also in those with congenital heart disease with Fontan physiology nearing the end of life. Prior to paracentesis, you should weigh the risks of circulatory collapse, especially in cardiac patients, and the need for albumin and electrolyte replacement.

Constipation and subsequent abdominal competition can be a major problem leading to shortness of breath for patients with neuromuscular disease, especially in infants with spinal muscular atrophy. Patients with muscle weakness and hypotonia usually require a daily bowel regimen. If constipated, they can have signs of severe respiratory distress. It is very important to be diligent about their bowel habits so as not to precipitate a respiratory crisis.

MUSCULOSKELETAL

Children with muscle weakness affecting their thoracic musculature and diaphragm can suffer from shortness of breath. Patients whose muscle weakness stems from a severe neurologic injury may not be able to report their subjective complaints. For this subset of patients, you should err on treating shortness of breath based on history and physical exam findings. Depending on patients' goals of care, they may want noninvasive positive pressure ventilation. These patients may also be faced with making the decision about tracheostomy and long-term mechanical ventilation.

CONCURRENT SYMPTOM-DIRECTED PHARMACOLOGIC MANAGEMENT

A provider working within the patient's stated goals of care should first attempt to treat or remove the primary source of the patient's dyspnea. While evaluation and treatment are underway, you should assess the patient's need for either short-term or long-term opioids for dyspnea relief. For patients whose goals are to prioritize comfort and symptom management, opioids are first-line treatment of dyspnea; opioids decrease the cognitive perception of air hunger and thus help stop or lessen the cycle of breathlessness and anxiety. You should initiate opioid therapy at 25–50% of normal starting doses, and for patients with hypotonia, consider starting even lower— perhaps 15–20% of normal starting doses. Some patients may also benefit from either as-needed or around-the-clock anxiolytic in conjunction with opioid therapy. Opioids and benzodiazepines used in combination are more effective than either opioids or benzodiazepines used alone, but combination therapy also carries increased risk for oversedation. When initiating opioid therapy, be mindful of expected side effects such as constipation and prescribe stimulant laxatives alongside your opioid prescription. Selective serotonin reuptake inhibitors (SSRIs) are helpful in patients with breathlessness and comorbid depression, but evidence is inconclusive if SSRIs are helpful for breathlessness alone.

NONPHARMACOLOGIC MEASURES FOR DYSPNEA MANAGEMENT

Patients often breathe easier sitting upright; most will prefer to sleep with the head of their bed elevated or propped on multiple pillows. For patients who are not hypoxemic, cooler temperatures in the room and a fan to the face may be helpful to relieve dyspnea without needing supplemental oxygen for comfort. It is believed that cool temperatures and a fan stimulate the skin and mucosa innervated by the trigeminal nerve to help "fool" the brain and reduce the sensation of breathlessness. Self-hypnosis empowers the patient with a tool to help calm the anxiety associated with dyspnea. Walking aids can help the patient conserve energy and thus decrease oxygen demand. Paced breathing and/or pursed-lip breathing are helpful tools to utilize during acute episodes of breathlessness. Cognitive–behavioral therapy and psychotherapy may be helpful to patients who are experiencing significant fear and anxiety associated with their breathlessness.

INTRACTABLE DYSPNEA

In some unfortunate cases, patients will suffer from intractable dyspnea at the end of life despite providers' best efforts to help them achieve comfort while maintaining their alertness to be able to enjoy their last hours to days. Palliative sedation can be offered to children suffering from intractable dyspnea. Continuous infusions of opioids and benzodiazepines are first-line agents to be used simultaneously. If needed, psychotropics such as pentobarbital should be considered, and in extreme cases, an anesthetic such a proprofol could be used.

PALLIATIVE TRACHEOSTOMIES

It is important to be mindful of potential biases, negative or positive, toward tracheostomies. For patients dealing with respiratory problems that are drastically impairing their quality of life, a tracheostomy could improve their quality of life and symptom burden. Although it is understood that tracheostomies require a significant amount of care, for some patients/families who are already familiar with noninvasive mechanical ventilation and airway clearance needs, a tracheostomy may not change their home routine significantly but could make the patient more comfortable. Tracheostomies should be approached on a case-by-case basis taking into consideration the patient's prognosis and goals of care.

CASE DISCUSSION

Our patient's source of dyspnea is irreversible. Because it is secondary to her bronchiolitis obliterans, all attempts to mitigate her symptoms with disease-directed therapy have been made with steroid bursts, immunotherapy, and inhaled medications. Her dyspnea was initially managed with extended-release morphine 15 mg by mouth twice daily. This improved her exercise tolerance enough so that she could get out of bed to a chair and ambulate with minimal assistance to the bathroom. She worked with the inpatient occupational therapist and child life specialist on breathing techniques and guided imagery to help her when she did have acute episodes of shortness of breath. She was discharged home with hospice care. Over the course of several weeks, her dyspnea worsened, her morphine dose was titrated up, and scheduled lorazepam was added. Eventually, her dyspnea became so severe and distressing that she was transitioned to a morphine continuous infusion and a midazolam continuous infusion and fortunately was able to achieve comfort with some good wakeful hours until her death.

KEY POINTS TO REMEMBER

- Dyspnea is the patient's subjective report of breathlessness and is not always associated with objective signs of respiratory distress (hypoxia, tachypnea, and retractions).
- Treatment options for dyspnea are guided by the etiology— reversible versus irreversible, patient's overall prognosis, and goals of care.
- First-line symptom management for dyspnea is opioids plus as-needed or scheduled benzodiazepines at 25–50% of normal starting doses.
- For patients with hypotonia and progressive muscle weakness, it may be safer to start at lower morphine doses such as 15– 20% of normal starting doses to reduce the risk of respiratory compromise.

Further Reading

Barbetta C, Currow DC, Johnson MJ. Non-opioid medications for the relief of chronic breathlessness: Current evidence. *Expert Rev Respir Med.* 2017;11(4):333–341.

Hauer JM. Treating dyspnea with morphine sulfate in nonverbal children with neurological impairment. *Pediatr Pulmonol.* 2015;50:E9–E12.

Pieper L, Zernikow B, Drake R, et al. Dyspnea in children with life-threatening and life-limiting complex chronic conditions. *J Palliat Med.* 2018;21(4):552–564.

Rowbottom L, Chan S, Zhang L, et al. Impact of dyspnea on advanced cancer patients referred to a palliative radiotherapy clinic. *Support Care Cancer.* 2017;25:2691–2696.

Spathis A, Booth S, Moffat C, et al. The breathing, thinking, functioning clinical model: A proposal to facilitate evidence-based breathlessness management in chronic respiratory disease. *Primary Care Respir Med.* 2017;27:27.

21 Why Isn't She Looking at Me?

Natalie Jacobowski

You visit a 2-year-old who is well known to
the palliative care team. She has a history of
developmental delay, pulmonary hypertension,
tracheostomy, and ventilator dependence. She has
been hospitalized for 2 months recovering from
tracheostomy while parents undergo teaching.
At baseline, she is nonverbal but interactive. She
developed acute infection 2 days ago. On examination,
she is writhing in bed, kicking herself, pulling her
hair and picking her ear to the point of bleeding, not
making eye contact, difficult to console, with nursing
at bedside trying to block her self-injurious behavior.
She does not respond to her name and is not soothed
by favorite toys or by repositioning to preferred
positions. Her nurse reports that she only sleeps
a few hours at night, is often awake and agitated
overnight, and sleeps more than usual during the day.
Attempts to treat pain with opioids and agitation with
benzodiazepines have not changed her symptoms.

What do you do now?

PEDIATRIC DELIRIUM

Pediatric delirium is an acute confusional state that is often reversible with treatment of the underlying cause and can be conceptualized as a state of acute brain dysfunction that can occur in patients during periods of acute and critical illness or at the end of life. It is a disturbance in attention, consciousness, cognition, and perception that often also commonly manifests with changes in sleep, behavior, emotions, and psychomotor activity. There is limited research on rates of pediatric delirium in palliative care. However, in adult palliative care patients, delirium has been identified in more than 90% of patients at the end of life and in more than 50% of adult patients admitted to a palliative care inpatient unit. Rates of delirium in pediatric patients have been most studied in the pediatric intensive care unit (PICU), where they range from 13% to 47% of patients. Accurate diagnosis of delirium can decrease both patient suffering and distress for families who witness their child with altered mental status because it allows delirium-focused treatment and avoidance of medications that can exacerbate delirium.

Delirium is defined by criteria in the fifth edition of the *Diagnostic and Statistical Manual of Mental Disorders* (DSM-5). The core features of delirium are outlined in Table 21.1. Delirium needs to be part of the differential diagnosis and assessment for patients with acute changes in mental status with concurrent acute illness or progression of illness at end of life. Overall, children with delirium are more similar to than different from

TABLE 21.1 **DSM-5 Criteria for Delirium**

Criteria 1	A disturbance in attention and awareness.
Criteria 2	Disturbance develops over a short period of time, is a change from baseline, and tends to fluctuate over the course of the day.
Criteria 3	An additional disturbance in cognition (e.g., memory deficit, disorientation, or disturbance in language, visuospatial ability, or perception).
Criteria 4	The disturbance is a direct physiological consequence of another medical condition, substance intoxication or withdrawal, exposure to a toxin, or due to multiple etiologies.

the more heavily studied population of adults with delirium. However, the following features are unique and more prevalent in pediatric delirium patients: increased mood lability, irritability, and anxiety. Therefore, consideration of delirium is warranted in pediatric patients who have these refractory symptoms that are not due to pain, other physical symptoms, or another primary psychiatric diagnosis. Regarding the patient presented in the case example, her worsened emotional lability, agitation, and lack of improvement despite treatment for pain and adequate treatment of respiratory distress and other physical symptoms raise concern for the potential presence of delirium. Upon consideration of the diagnostic criteria of delirium, her mental status change has been acute, and her nurses believe she has been less attentive and aware of her surroundings, which further warrants detailed delirium assessment.

To assess for delirium in this toddler, as in any patient, it is helpful to first know her baseline. This is especially relevant in young, nonverbal children or children with developmental delay. When possible, you want to know the child's baseline in terms of eye contact, smiling or reactions to preferred people and toys, ability to respond to commands/instructions, what usually helps console the child when distressed, and typical sleep/nap patterns. Table 21.2 outlines questions to ask about changes in behavior to assess for delirium in verbal and nonverbal pediatric patients. For your patient, at baseline she makes eye contact as well as smiles and claps her hands in response to preferred movies, songs, and interactions with staff. Nurses note that at baseline she will demonstrate some mild agitated behaviors such as kicking the side of the bed to get attention from nursing, but these behaviors cease when she gets the desired attention from staff. She has some chronic disruption in her sleep–wake cycle from a prolonged hospitalization of 2 months, but once asleep she tends to remain asleep without agitation. Since readmission to the cardiothoracic intensive care unit (CTICU), she has not demonstrated her usual smile or engagement with staff, her agitation is more extreme than ever before and does not cease with attention, her significant self-injury is new, and her physical and occupational therapists note that it is much more difficult to engage her in their sessions and keep her attention on an activity even when she is awake and not agitated. Based on this history, you now have even greater concern for delirium because this is an acute change from her baseline; she is demonstrating inattention; her

TABLE 21.2 Assessment of Mental Status and Potential Delirium in a Pediatric Patient

Core Features of Delirium	Assessment in Older/ Verbal Children	Assessment in Younger/ Nonverbal Children
Has there been an acute change in cognition? (Criterion 2 from DSM-5)	Obtain history from family/nurse. Fluctuation in past 24 hours.	Obtain history from family/nurse. Fluctuation in past 24 hours.
Is there evidence of disturbed attention or awareness? (Criterion 1 from DSM-5)	Serial 7 subtraction from 100 (five repetitions). Spell "world" backwards. Does the child remain engaged and attentive throughout interview?	Does the child make and maintain age-appropriate eye contact? Does the child consistently track an interesting visual stimulus?
Are there other disturbances in cognition? (Criterion 3 from DSM-5)	Does the child report auditory or visual hallucinations? Does the child have paranoia or other delusional thought? Does the child have impairment with orientation questions? Does the child demonstrate impaired memory? Does the child have psychomotor changes? Can the child follow two- or three-step commands (e.g. "Can you hold up two fingers, now a third finger?")?	Reaching for objects or appearing frightened by something seen but not actually present in the room (hallucinations). Lack of preferential response to familiar caregivers or favorite toys (impaired orientation). Impaired psychomotor or visuospatial skills such as difficulty putting pacifier to mouth to self-sooth Can child follow simple commands (e.g., point to nose)? Inconsolability and lack of response to usual methods for soothing and calming.

sleep–wake cycle is more disturbed; and although developmental delay and tracheostomy limit her communication, she is demonstrating cognitive impairment with lack of usual communication by smiles and gestures as well as increased irritability and inability to be consoled.

Delirium includes three main phenotypes: hyperactive, hypoactive, and mixed delirium. In hyperactive delirium, the patient often demonstrates increased agitation, restlessness, and emotional lability. These patients are often at greatest risk of harm such as self-extubation or removing their own intravenous catheters in the context of agitation and confusion. Because of this risk of self-harm, these patients often get the attention of the medical team. Hypoactive delirium patients typically demonstrate decreased responsiveness, apathy, and more withdrawn behavior. They have psychomotor slowing, are less interactive, and can at times appear as though acutely depressed until deficits in attention and cognition are further assessed to identify the presence of delirium. Because their symptoms do not cause the same disruption as hyperactive delirium, these patients can often be missed without routine screening or attention to delirium. Of concern is that more than 50% of these patients can have hallucinations and delusions, which contribute to acute distress during delirium but can also increase risk of post-traumatic symptoms after an episode of delirium. Mixed delirium is a combination of both hypoactive and hyperactive phenotypes. Despite being more clinically subtle, the most prevalent form of delirium is hypoactive delirium. In this patient case, she seems to primarily be presenting with hyperactive delirium given her high levels of agitation and extreme self-injurious behaviors.

To monitor mental status changes in pediatric patients, there are two primary screening tools that exist for screening for pediatric delirium. These screening tools were initially designed to be used in the PICU setting and to be used by nurses as an initial screen for possible presence of delirium. The Cornell Assessment of Pediatric Delirium (CAPD) is validated for patients from birth to age 18 years and is an observational screening tool that assesses eight domains of potential delirium symptoms. For patients with baseline developmental delays, their baseline score may be elevated and thus require contextual interpretation of their CAPD score that takes into account baseline functioning. Therefore, the screening instrument specifically asks about the presence or absence of developmental delays.

The Pediatric Confusion Assessment Method for the Intensive Care Unit (pCAM-ICU) and the Preschool Assessment Method for the Intensive Care Unit (psCAM-ICU) are designed as brief interactive screening tools to assess cognition and for potential delirium in pediatric patients aged 6 months to 18 years. For patients at higher risk of delirium, such as those in the ICU or those at the end of life who begin to show signs of delirium, it can be helpful to have these screening tools completed by trained providers ideally every shift, given the waxing and waning nature of delirium symptoms, to allow routine monitoring to detect changes in mental status that may otherwise be missed.

Once you are concerned for a potential diagnosis of delirium, there are two subsequent questions that should follow: What is the potential cause of the delirium? and How does this impact the patient's treatment? Because the first question partially informs the second, you begin by considering the potential causes of delirium.

Because delirium is due to an underlying medical illness or medication effect, the recognition of delirium inherently requires consideration of its cause. There are some predisposing risk factors that are more prevalent in many palliative care patients. Table 21.3 highlights predisposing

TABLE 21.3   **Risk Factors and Potential Causes of Delirium**

Predisposing Risk Factors for Delirium	Potential Causes of Delirium
Prior history of delirium	Acute infection
Cognitive impairment, developmental delay	Medications (especially anticholinergics, benzodiazepines, and opiates)
Neurological illness	Electrolyte abnormalities
Impaired communication (receptive [hearing and vision] or expressive [speech] communication)	Hypercarbia and hypoxia
Very young or very old age	Constipation and urinary retention
	Untreated/undertreated pain

factors that may increase a patient's risk of delirium as well as acute illness or medication effects that may be the cause of an episode of delirium. In your medically complex patient, as with many palliative care patients, the cause of delirium is often multifactorial. When considering those factors contributing to your patient's delirium, she has baseline risk factors of developmental delay, impaired communication, and difficulty maintaining her sleep–wake cycle as well as an acute infection, hypoxia at the time that symptoms began (which has since resolved), and recent polypharmacy with medications that can potentially contribute to delirium (she has received as-needed doses of lorazepam and morphine).

When considering the treatment for a patient with delirium, the primary treatment is treating the underlying cause of delirium. For palliative care patients, there are two additional questions involved in this process that require asking if the cause of delirium is reversible and if the interventions to treat the cause of delirium are within the goals of care for the patient. For example, the child in end-stage heart failure with delirium in his last days of life due to poor perfusion and progressive organ failure as part of the dying process does not have a reversible cause of delirium. At other times, the cause of the delirium may potentially be reversible, but the goals may not align with reversing the cause. Consider delirium in a teenager with end-stage cystic fibrosis with worsening respiratory status who has elected to pursue comfort care only and does not want inpatient admission, intravenous antibiotics, or noninvasive positive pressure ventilation. In this case, the focus is not interventions to attempt to reverse the hypoxia and hypercarbia driving the delirium but, rather, managing respiratory distress and symptoms of delirium. However, when possible and within the patient's goals of care, potentially reversible causes of delirium at all stages of illness should be explored and treated because delirium causes distress due to its symptoms but also by impairing a patient's ability to have alert, meaningful interactions.

When approaching treatment of delirium, in addition to addressing the underlying cause, there is an emphasis on nonpharmacologic interventions, simplifying polypharmacy as much as possible, and use of additional medication only as needed for symptoms. There are no US Food and Drug Administration-approved medications for treatment of delirium in children or adults, and the medications used to treat delirium help treat the symptoms of delirium but do not resolve the delirium. However, by helping to treat the agitation, they may provide some indirect treatment by allowing the ability to minimize use of medications such as opiates and benzodiazepines that further perpetuate the cycle of delirium. Table 21.4 highlights this framework for treatment of delirium.

Again, it is important to note that adding additional medication for delirium is toward the end of these treatment recommendations. However, there are times when treating the symptoms of delirium with medications is indicated (Table 21.5). You should more strongly consider treatment of symptoms when there is evidence of hallucinations, delusions,

TABLE 21.4 **Treatment of Delirium**

Treat underlying cause of delirium when able	For palliative care, consider: Is the cause reversible? Is treatment within goals of care?
Environmental interventions	Familiar objects and people at bedside Frequent reorientation Maintain routine and schedule (enlist child life specialists, physical therapist, and occupational therapist to assist) Provide vision/hearing aids if needed
Re-regulate sleep–wake cycle (including age-appropriate nap schedule)	Blinds open/lights on during the day Room dark at night and during nap time Cluster care as able during night/naps
Decrease potentially deliriogenic medications when able	Particular consideration to anticholinergic medications, benzodiazepines, and opiates
Use of psychotropic medications when needed	See Table 21.5

TABLE 21.5 Medications for Delirium Treatment

Medication	Benefit/Unique Features	Risk
Melatonin	Helps regulate sleep–wake cycle; theorized to treat one of the mechanisms of delirium	Minimal risk; occasionally cause increased nightmares in some patients
Alpha agonists (dexmedetomidine [Precedex])	Less deliriogenic medication for sedation in ICU; decreases hyperarousal and agitation; theorized to treat one of the mechanisms of delirium	Bradycardia and hypotension; collaborate with ICU physician
Quetiapine (Seroquel)—second-generation antipsychotic	Most published medication used in pediatric patients for delirium; most sedating (thus good if sleep very disturbed)	Sedating; lowest risk of EPS due to lower D_2 receptor affinity
Olanzapine (Zyprexa)—second-generation antipsychotic	Moderately sedating; effective antiemetic	Moderately sedating; moderate D_2 receptor affinity/EPS risk
Risperidone (Risperdal)—second-generation antipsychotic	Least sedating of second-generation antipsychotics	Higher D_2 receptor affinity/EPS risk (although usually well tolerated)
Haloperidol (Haldol)—first-generation antipsychotic	Available PO/IM/IV; able to give for acute agitation because available IV	Highest risk of EPS; risk of torsades when given IV (monitor ECG; monitor potassium and magnesium levels to decrease risk)

D_2, dopamine receptor subtype; ECG, electrocardiogram; EPS, extrapyramidal symptoms; ICU, intensive care unit; IM, intramuscularly; IV, intravenously; PO, orally.

disorganized thinking, agitation, hyperarousal, and sleep disturbance. For sleep disturbance, melatonin is a low-risk intervention to help re-regulate the sleep–wake cycle. For patients in the ICU setting who require sedation, dexmedetomidine, if hemodynamically tolerated, can potentially avoid or allow use of lower doses of opiates and benzodiazepines for sedation because these medications can be more deliriogenic. The most commonly used medications to treat symptoms of delirium are low-dose antipsychotics to target psychotic symptoms, agitation, and disorganized thinking. Antipsychotics are generally more beneficial for hyperactive delirium, and there are fewer data for use in hypoactive delirium unless target symptoms are prominently present. Second-generation antipsychotics are often chosen when a patient can tolerate an enteral medication because these medications have lower risk of extrapyramidal side effects such as dystonia related to lower degree of dopamine-2 receptor affinity. Haloperidol is a first-generation antipsychotic that is also effective and can be given intravenously, which is helpful when more rapid effect is needed. In reversible cases of delirium, benzodiazepines are not used because they can worsen confusion. However, for terminal delirium at the end of life when the cause is not reversible, benzodiazepines may be used to treat agitation and for their potential amnestic and muscle relaxation effects to meet a primary goal of giving a patient comfort at the end of life.

For our patient, you consider the previously mentioned multiple aspects of delirium treatment to determine her treatment plan. With regard to potential causes of delirium, she has a recent infection that is being treated, hypoxia that is now improved, and has had increased exposure to benzodiazepines and opiates for her agitation. The cause of delirium is likely reversible, and the goals of care are full intensive care intervention. Based on this, you identify that the underlying medical cause of her delirium (infection, associated hypoxia) has been addressed by the CTICU team. You recommend discontinuing benzodiazepines and only utilizing opioids if clear signs of pain with the hope of decreasing her exposure to deliriogenic medications. You talk with the CTICU about the importance of re-regulating the patient's day–night cycle, and her nurses work closely with child life, occupational therapy, and physical therapy to create a daily schedule and to keep the patient awake during the day other than naps to better facilitate sleep at night. Given the severity of agitation and her poor sleep at night, you start scheduled doses of quetiapine with as-needed doses available for agitation. During the next few days, her agitation progressively improves, and she begins to demonstrate improved eye contact, more frequent smiles, and her more typical behavior and interaction with staff. Once the patient reaches her baseline behavior and interactions with staff, you continue behavioral interventions but taper and discontinue her quetiapine dose over a few days because that medication is no longer needed for the acute agitation that was present during the episode of delirium.

KEY POINTS TO REMEMBER

- Delirium is an acute change in mental status with impaired attention and awareness due to a medical condition, medications, or combination of etiologies.
- Assessment of delirium in young children requires a developmental approach and assessing the child's baseline.
- Palliative care can assess causes of delirium and match treatment strategies with goals of care.
- Treating delirium includes treating the cause(s), environmental interventions, decreasing polypharmacy, and occasionally additional medication for delirium symptoms.

Further Reading

American Psychiatric Association. *Diagnostic and Statistical Manual of Mental Disorders*. 5th ed. Arlington, VA: American Psychiatric Publishing; 2013.

Hatherill S, Flisher AJ. Delirium in children and adolescents: A systematic review of the literature. *J Psychosom Res*. 2010;68:337–344.

Joyce C, Witcher R, Herrup E, et al. Evaluation of the safety of quetiapine in treating delirium in critically ill children: A retrospective review. *J Child Adolescent Psychopharmacol*. 2015;25(9):666–670.

Silver G, Kearney J, Traube C, Hertzig M. Delirium screening anchored in child development: The Cornell Assessment for Pediatric Delirium. *Palliat Support Care*. 2015;13(4):1005–1011.

Smith HA, Boyd J, Fuchs DC, et al. Diagnosing delirium in critically ill children: Validity and reliability of the Pediatric Confusion Assessment Method for the Intensive Care Unit. *Crit Care Med*. 2001;39(1):150–157.

Smith HA, Gangopadhyay M, Goben CM, et al. The Preschool Confusion Assessment method for the ICU: Valid and reliable delirium monitoring for critically ill infants and children. *Crit Care Med*. 2016;44(3):592–600.

Smith, HAB, Brink E, Fuchs DC, et al. Pediatric delirium monitoring and management in the pediatric intensive care unit. *Pediatr Clin North Am*. 2013;60:741–760.

Traube C, Silver G, Kearney J, et al. Cornell Assessment of Pediatric Delirium: A valid, rapid, observational tool for screening delirium in the PICU. *Crit Care Med*. 2014;42(3):656–663.

Traube C, Silver G, Reeder RW, et al. Delirium in critically ill children: An international point prevalence study. *Crit Care Med*. 2017;45(4):584–590.

Turkel SB, Hanft A. The pharmacologic management of delirium in children and adolescents. *Paediatr Drugs*. 2014;16(4):267–274.

22 The Lack of Movement

Billie Winegard

You are seeing an adolescent female for a hospital follow-up visit. She complains of nausea, abdominal pain, and decreased oral intake. Her history is significant for metastatic sarcoma. Recent scans showed progression of multiple bony lesions including her lumbar spine. Her surgical history is significant for a below the knee amputation approximately 2 months ago. She primarily uses her wheelchair to get around. She was discharged from the hospital 3 days ago after an admission for chemotherapy, which caused nausea and vomiting requiring antiemetics. She is currently taking ondansetron, oxycodone, and an acid blocker. She has been sleeping more. She had one small stool a week ago. Her family attributes this to not eating because she has no history of constipation. On exam, her abdomen is full and tender to palpation but soft with palpable hard stool. She has hypoactive bowel sounds. Rectal examination is deferred because she is neutropenic. Her neurologic exam is unremarkable.

What do you do now?

CONSTIPATION

Constipation is a common complaint in pediatrics, accounting for 3% of all visits to primary care physicians. It is a common cause of distress in children with serious illnesses and is one of the most common symptoms experienced by patients receiving palliative care. The risk for constipation increases as children near end of life, often causing significant pain, distress, and reduced quality of life.

Constipation can be difficult to define in pediatrics for many reasons. Constipation can mean different things to different individuals. There are wide variations in individuals' bowel habits—what is a normal frequency for some may be constipation for others, and the "normal" frequency of bowel movements changes at different ages. A suitable definition of constipation for children receiving palliative care is the passage of small, hard feces infrequently and with difficulty.

The most likely cause of the patient's symptoms in our case is constipation. She has many factors in her history that put her at risk, and her current complaints and physical exam are consistent with constipation. If there is doubt in the diagnosis of constipation, an abdominal radiograph may be performed to assess her stool burden or to rule out an obstruction.

The underlying cause of constipation in children receiving palliative care can vary widely. The most common cause of constipation in pediatrics is functional constipation—that is, constipation without an organic etiology. Given its high prevalence, it is very likely that many children referred to palliative care have functional constipation as a long-standing condition. Some children may have conditions that predispose them to constipation, such as cystic fibrosis, static encephalopathy, cerebral palsy, spinal cord trauma, or autonomic neuropathy. For children with cancer, constipation may be caused by a mechanical compression of the gut by a pelvic mass. Children with spinal cord tumors causing cord compression, hypothyroidism, electrolyte disturbances (hypercalcemia and hypokalemia), uremia, or intestinal obstruction should also be considered high risk for constipation. Changes in fluid and fiber intake as children's conditions advance may contribute to constipation. Many of the medications used by patients receiving palliative care can cause constipation, including chemotherapy, antacids, anticholinergics, antidepressants, opioids, sucralfate, sympathomimetics, antiemetics, and anticonvulsants. Contributing factors that may lead to stool withholding behaviors include limited privacy or access to a toilet or conditions that can cause pain with defecation, such as hemorrhoids or anal fissures.

For all patients with clinical concern for constipation, a thorough history should be obtained. This should include whether there is a history of constipation and treatments used in the past, in addition to current risk factors for constipation, including medications and diet. Frequency, consistency of stools, pain with stooling, and soiling should be gauged. Related symptoms should also be assessed, including abdominal pain, nausea, vomiting, and anorexia. Reports of diarrhea should not rule out constipation because it could represent obstipation with overflow. Urinary symptoms and numbness, weakness, and paresthesias of the lower extremities point to a possible spinal cord lesion that may require intervention if that is in line with the family's goals of care.

The physical exam should include both abdominal and neurologic evaluations. Abdominal palpation can elicit tenderness, and stool may be palpable. A rectal exam is recommended as part of the evaluation for constipation because it allows for assessment of rectal tone and causes of pain with stooling that may be contributing to withholding behaviors, such as anal fissures. If stool is present, a digital rectal exam allows for assessment of its consistency. However, a digital rectal exam is not always necessary to establish the diagnosis of constipation and should not be performed on neutropenic patients, such as children receiving chemotherapy, because it places them at risk for infection.

If the history reveals treatable causes of constipation, these should be addressed if possible. For those without a reversible cause, the goal should be prevention. Some simple interventions that can be implemented include establishing a regular bowel routine with access to a toilet and privacy, increasing physical activity to promote gut motility, and increasing fluid and dietary fiber.

In most cases, medications will be needed to prevent constipation (Table 22.1). The laxatives used in palliative care can be categorized according to their mode of action: softening, osmotic, stimulant, and others. Larger or more frequent doses may be required for evacuation or treatment, and

TABLE 22.1   **Medications Used in the Treatment of Constipation**

Class: Medication	Dose	Comments and Side Effects
Stool softener: docusate	Prophylaxis 10 times age in years = mg dose oral daily, divided up to four times per day; maximum dose 500 mg per day	May be administered via G-tube

Osmotic: lactulose	Prophylaxis
	  Ages 2–10 years: 2.5–7.5 ml oral daily
	  Ages >10 years: 15–30 ml oral daily
	Treatment
	  Ages <2 years: 2.5 ml oral twice a day
	  Ages 2–10 years: 2.5–7.5 ml oral twice a day
	  Ages >10 years: 15–30 ml oral twice a day
	Evacuation
	  Ages <2 years: 3 ml oral three times a day
	  Ages 2–10 years: 15–30 ml oral three times a day
	  Ages >10 years: 30 ml oral every 2 hours until patient has a bowel movement
		May be administered via G-tube
		Side effects
		Flatulence
		Abdominal cramps
		Bloating
		Diarrhea

Osmotic: polyethylene glycol	Prophylaxis
	  Ages 2–10 years: 8.5 g in 4 oz of liquid oral daily
	  Ages >10 years: 17 g in 8 oz of liquid oral daily
	Treatment
	  Ages 2–10 years: 8.5 g in 4 oz of liquid oral twice a day
	  Ages >10 years: 17 g in 8 oz of liquid oral twice a day
		May be administered via G-tube
		Requires a patient to take 4—8 oz of liquid
		Side effects
		Diarrhea
		Nausea
		Abdominal pain

Osmotic: magnesium citrate 1.745 g/30 ml solution	Evacuation
	  Ages <6 years: 2 ml/kg × 1 dose
	  Ages 6–12 years: 100 ml oral × 1 dose
	  Ages >12 years: 300 ml oral × 1 dose
		May be administered via G-tube

Class: Medication	Dose	Comments and Side Effects
Stimulant: senna 1.76 mg sennoside/ml 8.6 mg sennoside/tablet	Prophylaxis Ages <6 years: 2.5–5 ml or 1 tablet oral daily Ages 6–12 years: 2 tablets oral daily Ages > 12 years: 3 tablets oral daily Treatment Ages <6 years: 2.5–5 ml or 1 tablet oral twice a day Ages 6–12 years: 2 tablets oral twice a day Ages >12 years: 3 tablets oral twice a day Evacuation Ages <6 years: 30 ml or 6 tablets oral x 1 dose Ages 6–12 years: 45 ml or 9 tablets oral x 1 dose Ages >12 years: up to 90 ml or 18 tablets oral x 1 dose	May be administered via G-tube Also available as a tea Side effects Cramping Abdominal pain Nausea
Stimulant: bisacodyl	Evacuation Ages 6 months—2 years Suppository: 5 mg rectal daily Ages 2–12 years Oral tablet: 5 mg oral daily Suppository: 5–10 mg rectal daily Ages >12 years: Oral tablet: 5–15 mg oral daily Suppository: 10 mg rectal daily	Available as a tablet and suppository only Side effects Cramping Abdominal pain Nausea
Stimulant: glycerin Infant/pediatric: 1.2 g, 1.3 g Adult: 2 g, 2.1 g	Evacuation Ages <2 years: ½ infant/pediatric suppository rectal daily Ages 2–6 years: 1 infant/pediatric suppository rectal daily Ages >6 years: 1 adult suppository rectal daily	

G-tube, gastrostomy tube.

smaller or less frequent doses may be required for prophylaxis. Once evacuation is achieved, need for prophylaxis should be determined.

Softeners are often paired with a stimulant because they have limited efficacy on their own but can reduce pain associated with hard stools. Osmotic agents draw water into the intestinal lumen to hydrate and soften stools. These tend to be well tolerated with little cramping. Some require additional liquid (polyethylene glycol) and so should only be used when children can tolerate this fluid. Osmotic agents can cause diarrhea. If this occurs, the medication may be held until the diarrhea resolves and then the dose titrated until the child is having one or two soft stools daily. For infants older than age 1 month with constipation, 2–4 oz of 100% prune, pear, or apple juice can be given. The sugars in the juice are not well digested and act osmotically to draw fluid into the intestine to soften stool. Stimulant laxatives work on the mesenteric plexus to stimulate bowel motility. Other classes of medications that may be considered in palliative care patients are prokinetics such as erythromycin or metoclopramide for children with gastrointestinal hypoactivity. Suppositories and enemas work by softening stools or stimulating evacuation; as mentioned previously, the risk of infection and bleeding should be considered before these are used in patients with neutropenia or thrombocytopenia.

At times, constipation can be severe, and medications are insufficient to bring about evacuation. In these cases, manual disimpaction could be considered. Adequate analgesia and sedation should be provided as standard of care in pediatrics.

OPIOID-INDUCED CONSTIPATION

Children receiving opioids are at risk for opioid-induced constipation. Opioids reduce bowel motility and secretion and increase fluid absorption of the colon because stool spends more time moving through the colon. Unlike other side effects of opioids, opioid-induced constipation will not decrease with ongoing use. To prevent constipation, a regimen of laxatives for prophylaxis should be initiated at the time opioids are prescribed, with titration of doses to have a soft bowel movement every other day to up to twice daily.

Opioid antagonists can be used for opioid-induced constipation that is refractory to traditional laxatives. Studies in adults have shown that opioid antagonists can be effective in relieving opioid-induced constipation. Low-dose oral naloxone can be used. Oral administration theoretically takes advantage of hepatic metabolism, and so first-pass metabolism should prevent systemic effects and prevent withdrawal in patients who have a physiologic dependence. Ultra-low-dose intravenous administration may also be effective for constipation management.

A newer class of medications to treat opioid-induced constipation called peripherally acting μ-opioid receptor antagonists includes methylnaltrexone, naldemedine, and naloxegol. These drugs act by selectively blocking μ-opioid receptors in the gut to inhibit opioid-induced gastrointestinal hypomotility. Methylnaltrexone is available as a subcutaneous injection or tablet. Naldemedine and naloxegol are both tablets. The molecular structure of these medications prevents them from crossing the blood–brain barrier and interfering with central analgesia or triggering opioid withdrawal. Currently, there is no published information about dosing, safety, and efficacy for pediatric use for naldemedine and naloxegol. However, there are published reports of methylnaltrexone's effectiveness in pediatric patients, and the injection form contains weight-based dosing guidelines. Most patients who use methylnaltrexone have a bowel movement within 6 hours of administration. Injections can be given daily to every other day. The most common adverse effects are abdominal pain, flatulence, and nausea.

SUMMARY

In approaching end of life, constipation may become less important or cause less discomfort as other symptoms arise, and its management may become a lower priority. However, earlier in the disease course, it can cause significant discomfort. Because it is a very manageable symptom, care should be taken to treat it and prevent its recurrence.

- Constipation is a common and distressing symptom for children receiving palliative care.
- Prophylaxis may prevent constipation from becoming a significant problem, but it is frequently overlooked because other symptoms take priority.
- A bowel regimen should be co-prescribed with opioids as standard of care.
- Pairing a stimulant laxative with a stool softener or osmotic agent can be an effective combination to treat or prevent constipation.
- If opioid-induced constipation is refractory to traditional laxative regimens, there is literature that supports the efficacy of methylnaltrexone, a peripherally acting μ-opioid receptor antagonist, in inducing a bowel movement within a few hours of administration.

Further Reading

Anantharamu T, Sharma S, Gupta AK, Dahiya N, Singh Brashier DB, Sharma AK. Naloxegol: First oral peripherally acting mu opioid receptor antagonists for opioid-induced constipation. J Pharmacol Pharmacother. 2015;6(3):188–192.

Freidrichsdorf S, Drake R, Webster M. Gastrointestinal symptoms. In: Wolfe J, Hinds P, Sourkes B, eds. Textbook of Interdisciplinary Pediatric Palliative Care. Philadelphia: Elsevier; 2011:311–334.

Klaschik E, Nauck F, Ostgathe C. Constipation—modern laxative therapy. Support Care Cancer 2003;11(11):679–685.

Klick JC, Hauer J. Pediatric palliative care. Curr Probl Pediatr Adolesc Health Care 2010;40(6):120–151.

Madani S, Tsang L, Kamat D. Constipation in Children: A Practical Review. Pediatr Ann 2016;45(5):e189–e196.

Santucci G, Mack JW. Common gastrointestinal symptoms in pediatric palliative care: nausea, vomiting, constipation, anorexia, cachexia. Pediatr Clin North Am 2007;54(5):673–689, x.

Wolfe J, Grier HE, Klar N, et al. Symptoms and suffering at the end of life in children with cancer. N Engl J Med 2000;342(5):326–333.

23 Teenage "Bleh"

Dominic Moore and Colleen Marty

You are seeing a 17-year-old with recurrent osteosarcoma who reports feeling "bleh" during his third round of chemotherapy. He explains that he has not had energy to do what he enjoys, such as going to school and watching movies with friends.

Throughout treatment, he has kept up his typical teenage schedule. He enjoys online gaming with friends and pulled an all-nighter fueled by "energy drinks" when a new game was released. Because when he is gaming he is "back to his old self," his parents hesitate to set boundaries or limit this joy. On his chemotherapy regimen, he is transfusion dependent and receives packed red blood cells on a regular basis. He notes that he knows when he needs another transfusion because his energy is so low. When you ask about other symptoms, he acknowledges pain at the amputation site that is disturbing his sleep. Although he has oxycodone, he hesitates to use it because "I'm foggy enough as it is." He is willing to try other medication.

What do you do now?

FATIGUE

Fatigue resulting from illness may impact varied aspects of life and well-being for patients. The fatigue may have a mix of physical, mental, and emotional etiologies. These varied types of fatigue can touch upon all aspects of life for patients. Children and parents have both defined fatigue as a symptom that is common and distressing. The majority of parents and patients report that fatigue is present during their disease trajectory, and children with cancer have specifically identified fatigue as the symptom with the greatest impact on their quality of life.

Despite being a troubling symptom and area of interest for clinicians, fatigue has not been an area of robust investigation and publication. This chapter addresses considerations in presentation, diagnosis, and management of fatigue. Although there remains much to be learned, there is much that can be done for children struggling with this common symptom.

One of the first steps in recognizing fatigue in patients is a realization that it is, in fact, a problematic finding. Parents and providers often view fatigue as an integral and unavoidable part of the illness process, often recalling the last time they themselves were sick and how tired it made them. Providers may not be aware of validated tools for evaluation of fatigue, such as the Pediatric Quality of Life Inventory, the Childhood Fatigue Scale, and the Parent Fatigue Scale. Evaluation for fatigue, with or without these tools, is most helpful when administered serially. Because energy can wax and wane throughout the day, fatigue can easily be missed when a patient is evaluated during a period of higher energy.

Children reporting fatigue may focus on different aspects of the symptoms when talking with providers. Younger children often focus on the physical symptoms or feelings of fatigue. They may not be able to provide history on how their fatigue changes over the course of days or weeks, but they may talk about feeling tired or decline to engage in favorite activities. Older children and adolescents have been noted to focus on the way that fatigue impacts their life and goals. This might include an adolescent talking about difficulty in attending school, socializing with friends, or reaching goals in their personal life. They tend to be good historians, noting the time of day when symptoms are most severe and associations with other factors. One example is a patient undergoing treatment for cancer who may identify when fatigue is most severe in the cycle of treatment.

Parents find fatigue very distressing and may report their child withdrawing from family, daily routine, or beloved activities. If not specifically noted as fatigue, parents may report their children being more emotional than usual or having trouble with concentration, memory, and processing information. Parents are often excellent historians and may have a hypothesis for why the fatigue has gotten worse.

When the possibility of fatigue has been brought to a provider's attention, it is important to identify not only the impact of the symptom but also, when possible, the cause. Common and treatable factors for fatigue include anemia, medications, pain, disordered sleep, nutritional imbalance, changes in physical activity, emotional and/or spiritual distress, and medical comorbidities. Each of these underlying issues requires a different approach and has a different likelihood of response to therapy. For example, transfusions for anemia-related fatigue may be a great help depending on the setting in which they are given, but data related to efficacy of this treatment in children with advanced cancer have been limited and at times mixed.

Management of fatigue has no single, proven best approach. Each case should be evaluated separately, with a focus on treating the underlying cause of the fatigue when possible. An interdisciplinary approach is often required to fully address the factors contributing to a patient's fatigue. Nonpharmacologic approaches have been shown to be effective and may be used in concert with pharmacologic agents.

Sleep

Sleep is a basic requirement for functioning. Unfortunately, multiple aspects of caring for a sick child can compromise sleep for both the parent and the patient, and creating a restful environment can be challenging, diminishing both the quality and the duration of restorative sleep. The operational flow of a hospital, especially at night, may be a barrier to proper sleep hygiene. Healthy sleep practices include avoiding screen time, caffeine, and vigorous exercise in the 4 hours before sleep. In scheduling care, both in and out of the hospital, consideration should be given to clustering cares (including vital signs) to avoid frequently waking the patient. This practice can have the added benefit of providing adolescent patients a sense of control in an otherwise challenging situation. Additional tools to promote and provide structure to patients in and out of the hospital might include a consistent bedtime, elimination of unnecessary noise, and the presence of familiar objects.

Exercise

Exercise may seem counterintuitive for a patient who is already tired, but randomized control trials in adults have shown that exercise can decrease fatigue. In patients willing to consider physical activity, providers should consider involving physical therapy, occupational therapy, or providers specializing in physical medicine and rehabilitation. Starting with low-intensity exercises and increasing as possible can allow patients with limited physical abilities to engage in activities that may improve their function and energy.

Nutrition

Patients with life-limiting illness have various reasons for nutritional imbalance. For some of these patients, it is a lifelong issue. In every patient with fatigue, providers should search for deficiencies in calories, fluids, electrolytes, and intake. Simple interventions targeting these fundamental issues can have a significant impact on energy. It is noteworthy that the approach to these nutritional issues may differ at the end of life, at which time too much emphasis on nutrition can be misguided and even detrimental to the patient. When addressing and adjusting nutrition in patients with advanced illness, providers should be certain to keep patient and family goals in mind along with the overall trajectory of disease.

Integrative Therapies

Integrative therapies have been examined for fatigue, although large-scale studies are currently lacking. The most commonly discussed and recommended therapy is massage. Cognitive–behavioral therapy and guided imagery are two common and widely accepted modalities that have shown promise and should be considered. Patient interventions for managing stress and increasing relaxation may also yield benefit, especially in adolescent patients, who are acutely aware of the impact that their fatigue is having on the life they wish to live.

Pharmacologic Management

As is often the case, pharmacological studies in children are lacking, and we find ourselves looking to adult literature for information on treatment. Adult studies show methylphenidate to be a safe stimulant that may help with fatigue. There are case series examining the use of methylphenidate for fatigue in children, but to date, no randomized controlled trials have been performed. Pediatricians may be comfortable with methylphenidate because it is commonly used in primary care for behavioral management. Pediatricians should be mindful of the adverse effects of stimulant medication and prepare families for these issues before a stimulant is prescribed. This anticipatory guidance helps families appropriately interpret the signs that they see at home and in the health care setting. Corticosteroids and adenosine triphosphate infusions are other agents used in adults for fatigue, but the lack of available data in children make them less desirable options. Pharmacological management of fatigue may consist of "de-prescribing" or simplifying medication regimens. Certain medications or supplements may contribute to fatigue or negatively impact sleep hygiene even though they were initially prescribed for symptom management or even disease-directed therapy.

Education

Education for patients and families about fatigue can be helpful in the process of managing symptoms. It can also help establish realistic expectations and avoid unnecessary worry. It is important to consider discussing the clinical significance of fatigue in a patient's given setting. This discussion might help a family avoid worry when appropriate or help the family notice the signs that the medical team is observing. Helping families identify and anticipate behavior changes, especially irritability, can also help them understand that the root of the child's misbehavior is fatigue rather than unhappiness or family dysfunction. Data suggest that these simple instructions to parents can help improve processing and interaction.

Goals of Care

When considering the treatment of fatigue, the clinician should be sure to take into account patient and family goals in the context of current treatment. There are times when fatigue is a protection from interacting with the symptoms and pain associated with end of life. Treatment with stimulants or other interventions may unintentionally cause suffering or bring a patient to a state that is unacceptable to them or their family.

KEY POINTS TO REMEMBER

- Fatigue is a common and distressing symptom. Providers should be careful to screen for fatigue and be ready to address it.
- Consider the common causes of fatigue in your evaluation and tailor therapy accordingly.
- Providers should primarily use non-pharmacological therapies to treat fatigue.
- When pharmacological treatment is desired, methylphenidate is the agent of choice in children.
- Not all patients with fatigue require treatment

Further Reading

Blume ED, Balkin EM, Aiyagari R, et al. Parental perspectives on suffering and quality of life at end-of-life in children with advanced heart disease: An exploratory study. *Pediatr Crit Care Med*. 2014;15(4):336–342.

Huang IC, Anderson M, Gandhi P, et al. The relationships between fatigue, quality of life, and family impact among children with special health care needs. *J Pediatr Psychol*. 2013;38(7):722–731.

Miller E, Jacob E, Hockenberry MJ. Nausea, pain, fatigue, and multiple symptoms in hospitalized children with cancer. *Oncol Nurs Forum*. 2011;38(5):E382–E393.

Postovsky S, Lehavi A, Attias O, Hershman E. Easing of physical distress in pediatric cancer. In: Wolfe J, Jones BL, Kreicbergs U, Jankovic M, eds. *Palliative Care in Pediatric Oncology*. Cham, Switzerland: Springer; 2018:119–157.

Tomlinson D, Diorio C, Beyene J, Sung L. Effect of exercise on cancer-related fatigue: A meta-analysis. *Am J Phys Med Rehabil*. 2014;93(8):675–686.

Varni JW, Burwinkle TM, Katz ER, Meeske K, Dickinson P. The PedsQL in pediatric cancer: Reliability and validity of the Pediatric Quality of Life Inventory Generic Core Scales, Multidimensional Fatigue Scale, and Cancer Module. *Cancer*. 2002;94(7):2090–2106686.

Wolfe J, Hinds P, Sourkes B. *Textbook of Interdisciplinary Pediatric Palliative Care*. Philadelphia, PA: Elsevier; 2011.

24 A Sad Side Effect of Cancer

Laura Rose Musheno

You are the palliative care physician seeing in follow-up a 16-year-old young man with relapsed, metastatic osteosarcoma that has continued to progress despite treatment. His oncologist has told him and his family that his prognosis is likely weeks to months. His mother pulls you aside before you enter the room to share that she is very worried about her son. She tells you that he has become increasingly withdrawn, now refusing visits from friends and family. He does not seem to enjoy any activities that he once used to, and he expressed to her the other day that he feels guilty for being a burden to his family. You speak with the patient alone and ask him how he has been feeling. He shares that he feels sad most of the time and worthless to his family and friends. As he continues to open up to you, you contemplate his diagnosis and potential treatment options.

What do you do now?

DEPRESSION

Depression is a serious diagnosis that disproportionately affects patients with advanced illness. Studies have revealed that as many as 15% of cancer patients have been diagnosed with depression, a rate that is approximately three times that of the general population. Adolescents and young adults with advanced illness are at even higher risk of depression, grappling with life-threatening disease alongside the usual challenges of emerging adulthood. Unfortunately, depression is frequently underrecognized in patients with advanced illness because the nuances of diagnosis in this population can make it more difficult for clinicians to identify. However, it is imperative to diagnose and treat depression promptly because it can have a devastating impact if left untreated. Depression in patients with serious illness has been shown to be highly associated with poorer quality of life (for both patients and their caregivers), higher symptom burden, decreased adherence to treatment, and, most significantly, increased mortality.

Although depression is certainly prevalent in patients with advanced illness, there is a common misconception that it is a "normal" reaction for patients who have been diagnosed with a life-limiting disease. Many patients have this misconception as well. However, not all, or even most, terminally ill patients are depressed, and thus it should not be considered the norm. When caring for these patients, it is important to differentiate pathological depression from normal anticipatory grief that often occurs when diagnosed with a life-limiting disease. Anticipatory or preparatory grief refers to the process of grieving an impending loss. Patients may grieve a variety of losses after diagnosis with a serious illness—from physical (loss of physical strength) to social (changing relationships with friends or family) and emotional and spiritual (loss of purpose or faith). Patients may also begin to prepare for the anticipated loss of their own life as well. A number of features can help a clinician distinguish between anticipatory grief and depression. Although patients do inevitably experience feelings of sadness when they grieve, these feelings wax and wane over time. Patients may express having both good and bad days, but they are still able to find joy in life, enjoying times with friends and family. In contrast, for patients with depression, the sadness is much more persistent and usually associated with negative feelings of self-worth. They have difficulty finding pleasure in activities that they once used to enjoy, and they may isolate themselves from friends and family. Feelings of guilt can be overwhelming in those who are depressed. Although these nuances can be difficult to distinguish, often the answer becomes clearer when providers start the conversation, allowing space for patients to open up about their feelings.

Making a diagnosis of depression in pediatric patients with advanced illness can be challenging for a variety of reasons. There are several screening tools for major depression used in the primary care setting, one of the most common being the Patient Health Questionnaire (PHQ), which has a modified version for adolescents. However, these screening tools are not always as effective in identifying depression in patients with serious illnesses. These tools often focus on somatic symptoms of depression that often occur as a result of their underlying disease, such as decreased appetite, fatigue, and altered sleep. Therefore, in adolescents and young adults suspected to be depressed, it is often more helpful to focus on the psychological symptoms, such as anhedonia, social withdrawal, and feelings of worthlessness, hopelessness, and guilt. In contrast, it is important to note that younger children with depression and serious illness can be even more perplexing to diagnose because they more often present with heightened somatic symptoms as well as increased irritability, rather than depressed mood.

Once depression is recognized, it is important to begin treatment quickly given the significant impact on morbidity and mortality. Before considering disease-specific treatment options for depression, first evaluate for any confounding physical symptoms or reversible medical causes. Uncontrolled pain, for example, has been found to be associated with higher rates of depression in cancer patients. Although providers should not delay treatment specific for depression, they must recognize the effect that poorly controlled pain, dyspnea, nausea, or insomnia may have on a patient's well-being and optimize treatments directed toward those symptoms as well. Moreover, as with any patient presenting with a psychiatric symptom, providers should evaluate for potentially reversible organic causes. Many patients with advanced illness are on a number of medications, some of which can have the unwanted side effect of depressed mood. Glucocorticoids, opioids, benzodiazepines, and certain chemotherapeutic agents can all be potential offenders. It is worth reviewing the patient's medication list and having a conversation with the primary treatment team about whether any of these medications can be adjusted or discontinued if thought to be contributing.

Depression treatment requires a multimodal and multidisciplinary approach. Although there are a number of pharmacologic treatment options, nonpharmacologic strategies are just as, if not more, important for the treatment of depression in this population. Providers should strongly consider referral to counseling because engaging patients in cognitive–behavioral therapy has been shown to be an effective treatment, often used in conjunction with medications. Children may more easily open up when engaging in play therapy or with an art or music therapist. Adolescents may find value in completing legacy-building activities. The members of the interdisciplinary palliative care team can also be a valuable resource to help support these patients. Social workers can often be a source of emotional support, particularly if there are complex social dynamics and stressors. Patients who express spiritual and existential distress may benefit from chaplain support. Although these modalities have not been rigorously studied for efficacy, alternative therapies such as aromatherapy, massage, hypnosis, or reiki may have a positive and calming effect for some patients.

Because more medications have become available for depression treatment that are better tolerated and with less side effects, clinicians should have a low threshold for starting a medication for depression. There are a number of categories of medications available for the adult population, many of which are available for children and adolescents as well. The first consideration when choosing a medication for depression in a patient with a life-limiting illness is the patient's prognosis. Many antidepressants used in the general population do not take effect for at least 6–8 weeks. This is problematic because patients with a shorter prognosis may not live long enough to derive any benefit from these medications. A general rule of thumb to follow is that for patients who have a prognosis of 2 months or less, stimulant medications are recommended for treatment, whereas if prognosis is more than 2 months, antidepressants are recommended. Clinicians can also consider initiating treatment with a stimulant in addition to an antidepressant for patients with a longer prognosis and severe depression necessitating more immediate treatment.

Psychostimulants are a better option for patients with depression and a more limited prognosis because they have a much quicker onset, often having a therapeutic effect within 48 hours. Although they may not be as effective as antidepressants, studies have shown that they are reasonably beneficial for depression and have a positive effect on mood. The most common psychostimulants used are methylphenidate and modafinil. They are both available by mouth. Adverse effects to psychostimulant medications include increased blood pressure and heart rate. Thus, in patients with cardiovascular disease, risks and benefits for each patient must be carefully evaluated prior to initiating treatment. They also have the potential to worsen delirium as well as suppress appetite. It is worth mentioning that ketamine, an N-methyl-D-aspartic acid receptor antagonist currently used in the palliative care setting as an adjuvant treatment for pain, may also have some use as a rapidly acting antidepressant. Although evidence is currently limited to small trials and case studies, the data are promising that this may be an effective treatment for severe depression that is deserving of further evaluation in larger scale randomized controlled studies.

The primary classes of antidepressants defined based on their mechanism of action are selective serotonin reuptake inhibitors (SSRIs), serotonin–norepinephrine reuptake inhibitors (SNRIs), and tricyclic antidepressants (TCAs). There are also some atypical antidepressants that do not fit into these general categories. Generally, no one class of antidepressants has been found to be more effective than another, and this is true as well for medications within a particular class. When reviewing treatment options, choose a medication with the lowest side effect profile or with additional properties that may be beneficial for your patient's other symptoms or comorbidities. It may be helpful to engage a child and adolescent psychiatrist for assistance in determining the best treatment option. Clinicians should also refer to psychiatry sooner if the patient has a previous history of mental illness, has failed first-line therapy, or has suicidal ideation.

SSRIs are the most commonly prescribed class of antidepressants because they are both effective and well tolerated. Some of the commonly used SSRIs are citalopram, sertraline, fluoxetine, escitalopram, and paroxetine. SSRIs can be a good choice in patients with comorbid anxiety as well. Although they are usually well tolerated, they can have side effects including gastrointestinal upset, sexual dysfunction, as well as QT-interval prolongation on electrocardiogram. Most of these agents have a predisposition for being more activating and therefore can contribute to insomnia, except for paroxetine, which tends to be more sedating. When discontinued abruptly, some of these medications can cause withdrawal symptoms; therefore, it is important to caution patients and families not to discontinue them abruptly. All of these agents are administered once daily and available as both a tablet and a liquid formulation.

Not only are SNRIs effective as a treatment for depression but also, because serotonin and norepinephrine are both neurotransmitters involved in pain transmission, they have been shown to be effective for the treatment of neuropathic pain as well. SNRIs include duloxetine and venlafaxine. These agents also have a favorable side effect profile, with side effects similar to those of SSRIs, and therefore are also often used as first-line agents for depression.

TCAs are the oldest class of antidepressants and are less commonly used due to their side effect profile. Their anticholinergic and sedative side effects often limit their use. They also have the potential for QT prolongation. Although they do have more potential for toxicity, they can be useful for patients who have comorbid neuropathic pain or insomnia. Amitriptyline and nortriptyline are the most commonly used TCAs. Both are given by mouth, and they are often dosed at nighttime because they are sedating. Nortriptyline may be better tolerated because it typically has fewer anticholinergic side effects.

Some of the other antidepressants used that do not fit into the previously discussed categories include mirtazapine, which can be both sedating and increase appetite and therefore is a potential option in a depressed patient who also has difficulty sleeping or decreased appetite. Bupropion is a serotonin, norepinephrine, and dopamine reuptake inhibitor that is more activating than other depressants. However, it does have the potential to lower the seizure threshold.

SUMMARY

The importance of recognizing and treating depression, especially in young patients with advanced illness, cannot be understated. Although it can be difficult to diagnose, when depression is appropriately treated, this can help alleviate a significant contributor to suffering for these patients. Providers should have a high index of suspicion for depression in patients with serious illness and a low threshold to initiate treatment.

KEY POINTS TO REMEMBER

- Depression is common in patients with advanced disease, and it is important to promptly recognize and treat due to its deleterious effects on quality of life.
- Grief is a common reaction in patients with life-limiting illnesses, and it should be differentiated from depression.
- Psychostimulants should be used to treat patients with a shorter prognosis, whereas antidepressants should be standard in those likely to live more than a few months.

Further Reading

Block S. Assessing and managing depression in the terminally ill patient. *Ann Intern Med.* 2000;132(3):209.

Coughtrey A, Millington A, Bennett S, et al. The effectiveness of psychosocial interventions for psychological outcomes in pediatric oncology: A systematic review. *J Pain Symptom Manage.* 2018;55(3), pp. 1004–1017.

Grotmol K, Lie H, Hjermstad M, et al. Depression—A major contributor to poor quality of life in patients with advanced cancer. *J Pain Symptom Manage.* 2017;54(6):889–897.

Lloyd-Williams M, Spiller J, Ward J. Which depression screening tools should be used in palliative care? *Palliat Med.* 2003;17(1):40–43.

Park E, Rosenstein D. Depression in adolescents and young adults with cancer. *Dialogues Clin Neurosci.* 2015;17(2):171–180.

Periyakoil V. Fast facts and concepts #43: Is it grief or depression? 2019. Retrieved February 14, 2019, from https://www.mypcnow.org/blank-rc5hu

Quill T, Bower K, Holloway R, et al. *Primer of Palliative Care.* 6th ed. Chicago, IL: American Academy of Hospice and Palliative Medicine; 2014:100–109, 232–233.

25 My Patient Is Twitching; Could It Be Itching?

Alexis Morvant and Emma Jones

You are seeing a 12-year-old male with osteosarcoma localized to the right femur. He has been receiving high-dose chemotherapy with good local response and is now admitted for surgical resection with limb salvage operation. He was healthy prior to his cancer diagnosis. He experienced severe nausea with initial rounds of chemotherapy, and his mother describes him as "very sensitive to side effects." His mood has been somewhat poor, which his mother believes is "to be expected."

On postoperative day 1, you visit to assess his pain control. He is receiving morphine via patient-controlled analgesia (PCA) pump, and he reports his pain is well controlled. He reports no other side effects. You notice he is fidgeting in bed and see scratch marks on his face. When questioned about itching, he reports that this has been a problem all night and has kept him from sleeping well. He is otherwise alert and oriented. Physical exam of the skin reveals no rash or other abnormality.

What do you do now?

OPIOID-INDUCED PRURITUS

Pruritus is a known adverse effect of opioid therapy. It occurs in 2–10% of patients receiving systemic opioid therapy. Incidence may be even higher in those receiving neuraxial (epidural and intrathecal) opioids. This symptom is often reported as extremely distressing and often more troublesome than the pain itself. As in the case of your patient, patients may perceive a general unease or restlessness, and it is essential to ask about the presence of itching. Younger patients may lack the vocabulary to describe the sensation but will be observed to be restless, scratching, or generally irritable despite adequate pain control. In very young children, it may be difficult to assess if such nonspecific symptoms are due to pruritus or another cause, and it is wise to keep this in the differential of any patient on opioid therapy.

The mechanism of opioid-induced pruritus is not completely understood; however, the current model involves a mix of a small contribution of peripheral fibers and larger contribution of central impulses. Peripherally, the sensation of itch is transmitted from the skin via C-nociceptors, or C-type nerve fibers. These fibers transmit itch signal to the dorsal horn of the spinal cord and eventually make their way to the somatosensory cortex. Morphine may stimulate non-immunological histamine release from mast cells in the dermis, which will be transmitted via these C-fibers as itch. This pathway will be diminished using antihistamines. Itch sensation may also be generated by direct stimulation of receptors in the dorsal horn of the spinal cord. This pathway is diminished by opioid antagonists and is not affected by antihistamines. In addition, there is empiric evidence for use of dopamine (D_2), serotonin ($5\text{-}HT_3$), and prostaglandin receptor antagonists, suggesting that these receptors also play a role in the generation of itch sensation.

Given this complex pathophysiology and relatively scant evidence, the treatment of pruritus in pediatric palliative care is very empiric. It would be reasonable to start with a trial of antihistamine medication because these agents are widely used and general clinician comfort level is high. It is likely in many cases that any observed benefit is due to sedation and not direct relief of itch sensation.

Use of opioid antagonists is more likely to directly address the causative mechanism and provide relief while awake. Nalbuphine, which is a

> BOX 25.1 **Medications for Opioid-Induced Pruritus**
>
> Naloxone 0.25–2 mcg/kg/hour
> Nalbuphine 0.01–0.02 mg/kg (1.5 mg max) IV every 6 hours prn
> Ondansetron 0.15 mg/kg (max 8 mg) po/IV every 8 hours prn

mixed opioid agonist–antagonist, is given as intravenous (IV) intermittent dosing on an as-needed basis. Naloxone is a pure opioid antagonist and is frequently used for rapid reversal in the setting of overdose. When used at a very low dose, naloxone can provide just enough antagonism to resolve pruritus. Due to a short half-life, naloxone must be given as a continuous infusion to be most effective. See Box 25.1 for dosing.

Opioid Rotation

Rotation from one opioid to another is a common and often effective strategy for overcoming side effects. In one study of PCA usage in opioid-naive patients aged 4–13 years, pruritus was the reason for rotation in 65% of the cases; however, the need for rotation was overall very low (only 26 of 514 cases). Morphine is often the drug of choice for initiating opioid therapy and therefore the most likely to be rotated "away from." Morphine is also known to induce histamine release and hydromorphone does not, suggesting a potential advantage in diminishing pruritus. Propensity to induce pruritus is not a reason to suggest selection of one opioid over another; however, there is evidence to support the rotation to another opioid if a patient develops pruritus.

Antihistamines

First-generation histamine (H1) blockers include hydroxyzine, diphenhydramine, cyproheptadine, and promethazine. Because these agents readily penetrate the central nervous system and have additional receptor activity (antimuscarinic, α-adrenergic, and serotonin), sedation is a common side effect. Second-generation H1 blockers, such as cetirizine and fexofenadine, have less central nervous system penetration and more specific H1 binding, thus reducing significant side effects. In a study of patients with chronic urticaria, there was no significant difference in efficacy between hydroxyzine and cetirizine. This suggests that use of the less sedating second-generation agents is preferred. Box 25.2 lists diseases that respond to antihistamine therapy.

Psychological or Emotional Strategies

The itch center in the brain is located near to emotion processing centers, and therefore the sensation of itch can be experienced on a more emotional level. In addition, disrupted sleep and constant discomfort can deplete patients' coping abilities. Psychosocial support and use of nonpharmacologic therapies are essential to providing comprehensive pruritus management.

General Management Strategies

Skin integrity is one of the most important steps to pruritus management. Attempting to moisturize skin and keeping the environment cool and humidified are helpful strategies. Dry skin can be a culprit and can exacerbate pruritus no matter the cause. Topical therapies such as cooling agents, corticosteroids, and antihistamines can be an initial approach after improving skin integrity and the environment. Cool compresses, emollients, and topical menthol may all be immediately soothing.

Nonpharmacologic Treatments

Child life therapists may assist with providing distracting or calming age-appropriate activities, and many are skilled in guided imagery and mindfulness exercises as well. Integrative therapies such as reiki, hypnosis, aromatherapy, or massage may also be beneficial.

Reassurance and counseling about the treatment plan and time frame of medication efficacy will allow the team to align with the patient and family. Ensuring that the patient knows their concerns are being addressed is also important.

Your 12-year-old patient received one dose of diphenhydramine and fell asleep. He continued to scratch his face and arms even while asleep, and the team decided to initiate a naloxone infusion. Within 2 hours of naloxone infusion, he reported complete relief of his itch and his mood was visibly improved. During the next 5 days, his PCA usage diminished, and he was transitioned to oral morphine for discharge. Naloxone infusion was discontinued with no return of pruritus. This phenomenon is often observed and suggests that pruritus is somewhat dose and route dependent. In addition, patients appear to develop tolerance to pruritus after 3 or 4 days of opioid use.

OTHER CAUSES OF PRURITUS

Uremic pruritus: Uremia causes pruritus in multifactorial mechanisms partly due to skin dryness in addition to abnormal mast cell proliferation and accumulation of metabolites. Medications to consider in uremic pruritus: μ-opioid antagonists (naloxone and naltrexone), 5-HT$_3$ receptor antagonist (ondansetron), and antidepressants (paroxetine, sertraline, and mirtazapine).

Cholestasis: The mechanism by which patients experience pruritus due to liver dysfunction is thought to be from cholestasis, although there is no consensus on the exact pathophysiology. The amount of bilirubin in the blood does not directly correlate with the intensity of pruritus. Both central and peripheral mechanisms are involved, and a diverse, empiric approach is key for management of pruritus in liver dysfunction. Medications to consider in cholestatic pruritus: μ-opioid antagonist (naloxone), 5-HT$_3$ (ondansetron), antidepressants (paroxetine, sertraline, and mirtazapine), pregnane X receptor antagonist (rifampin), and bile acid sequestrants (cholestyramine and colestipol).

Malignancy: Children with oncologic disorders can also experience pruritus outside of organ dysfunction. In general, pruritus is more common in leukemias and lymphomas than solid tumors. Also, children can get skin metastasis in addition to nerve entrapment that can be additional causes of pruritus. Of course, remember that many patients with cancer also experience cancer-related pain and are supported with opioids. Keep opioid-induced pruritus high on the differential for patients who have pruritus and cancer.

Medications to consider using in patients with pruritus associated with malignancy:

Lymphoma—glucocorticoids (dexamethasone and prednisone)

Other malignancies—antidepressants (paroxetine, sertraline, and mirtazapine), NK1 receptor antagonist (aprepitant)

Neuropathic-induced pruritus secondary to tumor impingement—gabapentenoids (gabapentin and pregabalin).

Box 25.3 lists systemic diseases that may have associated pruritus, and Box 25.4 lists medications that can induce pruritus.

BOX 25.3 **Systemic Diseases with Associated Pruritus**

Renal: chronic renal failure

Hepatic: primary biliary cirrhosis, cholestasis, and hepatitis

Hematologic: polycythemia vera, lymphoma, and iron deficiency

Endocrine: hyperthyroidism, hypothyroidism, carcinoid syndrome, and diabetes mellitus

Miscellaneous: AIDS, multiple sclerosis, central nervous system tumors, drugs, and psychosis

---

Opioids

Angiotensin-converting enzyme inhibitors

Common tumor modulating medications

  BRAF inhibitors (vemurafenib)

  Epidermal growth factor inhibitors (cetuximab, erlotinib, and
    panitumumab)

Any drug that was started just prior to the start of the itching

OTHER POTENTIAL AGENTS TO CONSIDER

Gabapentin and pregabalin are γ-aminobutyric acid analogs. They were initially created as antiepileptics and have since been found to have a wide use outside of epilepsy. Gabapentin seems to work centrally by inhibiting pruritus perception in addition to minimizing action potentials in spinal neurons. Ultimately, gabapentin helps inhibit transmission of nociceptive sensations to the brain and at the same time suppresses pruritus sensation. Gabapentin can be used for multiple indications, such as uremia, malignancy, neurologically induced causes, and idiopathic causes. Gabapentin and pregabalin are usually well tolerated; the most common side effects are somnolence, vertigo, and fatigue. Gabapentin is renally cleared, so use with caution with kidney dysfunction, especially at the time of discontinuing dialysis.

Ondansetron is an antagonist at 5-HT_3 serotonin subtype receptors. It can be helpful for opioid-induced pruritus. Studies are minimally compelling that ondansetron is helpful for cholestasis pruritus or uremic pruritus, but with the low side effect profile, it can be used.

Topical capsaicin is an alkaloid found in the nightshade plant family. It targets transient receptor potentials, which help with perception of pruritus by activating pain neurons by releasing substance P. It seems to be particularly helpful in uremic pruritus and neuro-induced pruritus.

Menthol and camphor help attend to pruritus by providing a cooling effect that can confuse neurons to forget about the pruritus feeling. These have been shown to be useful in some patients, especially those with a rash present.

BOX 25.5 **Less Common Pharmacologic Agents That May Be Used for Pruritus**

Paroxetine
Thalidomide
Doxepin
Mirtazapine
Sertraline
Tacrolimus (topical)

Lidocaine delivered by a patch or topical cream can be helpful especially for neuropathic pruritus. One must keep in mind that in large quantities, lidocaine can cause methemoglobinemia in infants and small children.

Corticosteroids and diphenhydramine creams can be helpful when there is skin inflammation at the site such as contact dermatitis.

Other less common agents to consider using are shown in Box 25.5.

KEY POINTS TO REMEMBER

- Pruritus management is empiric without expansive evidence-based approaches. Thus, it is important to develop a stepwise management style when attending to pruritus in the seriously ill population.
- When opioid-induced pruritus is suspected, consider opioid antagonist or opioid rotation. One can also consider antihistamine, which most likely works as sedation rather than mechanistically easing pruritus.
- When thinking about pruritus in the seriously ill population, do not forget nonpharmacologic interventions such as hypnosis, guided imagery, Reiki, cool packs, and child life therapists to help with distraction.

Further Reading
Anand, S. Gabapentin for pruritus in palliative care. *Am J Hosp Palliat Care.* 2013;30(2):192–196.

Bunchorntavakul C, Reddy KR. Pruritus in chronic cholestatic liver disease. *Clin Liver Dis.* 2012;16:331.

Dalal S. Palliative care: Overview of pruritus and sweating. UpToDate; 2019. Retrieved from https://www.uptodate.com/contents/palliative-care-overview-of-pruritus-and-sweating/contributors

DiGiusto M, Bhalla T, Martin D, Foerschler D, Jones M, Tobias J. Patient-controlled analgesia in the pediatric population: Morphine versus hydromorphone. *J Pain Res.* 2014;7:471–475.

O'Donoghue M, Tharp M. Antihistamines and their role as antipruritics. *Dermatologic Ther.* 2005;18:333–340.

PDQ Cancer Information Summaries. Pruritus PDQ. Retrieved January 15, 2019, from https://www.cancer.gov/about-cancer/treatment/side-effects/skin-nail-changes/pruritus-hp-pdq

Reich A, Szepietowski JC. Opioid-induced pruritus: An update. *Clin Exp Dermatol.* 2009;35:2–6.

Siemens W, Xander C, Meerpohl JJ, Antes G, Becker G. Drug treatments for pruritus in adult palliative care. *Dtsch Arztebl Int.* 2014;111:863–870.

Siemens W, Xander C, Meerpohl JJ, Buroh S, Antes G, Schwarzer G, Becker G. Pharmacological interventions for pruritus in adult palliative care patients. *Cochrane Database Syst Rev.* 2016;2016(11):CD008320.

26 Is My Baby Feeling Hungry?

Lindsay B. Ragsdale

You are at the bedside of a 2-day-old neonate in the neonatal intensive care unit (NICU) who was just diagnosed with a lethal skeletal dysplasia that is characterized by shortened and deformed long bones and a tiny rib cage with severe pulmonary hypoplasia. The infant is in distress even on maximal mechanical ventilation, and the parents, after learning about the prognosis associated with this skeletal dysplasia, do not want to prolong their daughter's suffering and ask to discontinue life support. After discontinuing the ventilator, the infant's oxygen saturations are in the 40s, and she is cyanotic but comfortable. The father looks at you with tears in his eyes and asks if his daughter is feeling hungry because she is not currently being given feeds.

What do you do now?

MANAGING FEEDS AND FLUIDS AT END OF LIFE

Bearing witness to a child dying is an emotionally charged time for family and the staff. During this time period, many questions can arise about what the child is experiencing and what can be done to relieve suffering. Providing nutrition to children is an innate instinct for parents and is a way many parents show love and connection to their children. Not being able to provide nutrition can be difficult for families, and they may worry about hunger pains or feelings of starvation. Reassurance about the natural shutdown process of the body and explanations about lack of hunger or satiety can be helpful to calm fears. In some cases, providing artificial nutrition and hydration (ANH) to a patient who is dying can cause harm and suffering. Exploring these topics with families can be helpful to guide them through this heartbreaking time.

Infants and children need assistance with feeding as part of their natural developmental growth with breastfeeding, bottles, spoon feeds, small finger foods, and prepared meals. Being responsible for the child's nutrition is part of our duty and responsibility as caregivers. When we are no longer able to accomplish this duty, many parents worry about failing to provide for their child or being a "bad" parent. Our job is to help the family understand what is happening with their child's body and work together to develop the best strategy to care for the child. Often, this involves reassurance and explanation to the family about the process but also to directly address their fears and perception of duty to their child.

Diseases that affect the abdomen can have a direct effect on the ability to tolerate feeds. Intestinal perforation, masses, obstruction, and ischemia are all common causes of gut failure at end of life in children and can be reasons that feeds will not be tolerated. The natural dying process can lead to declining body functioning in which oxygen levels drop, lactate increases, electrolytes change, organs shut down, and the body readjusts to a declining metabolic state. If ANH is added during the acute dying phase, the body may not be able to adequately handle the volume or osmotic load and can start to leak fluid into the tissues, lungs, and abdomen. This third spacing of extra fluid can cause respiratory distress, dyspnea, peripheral edema, and ascites, which will add to the suffering of the patient. Often, if these downstream effects of ANH are explained, parents understand and agree not to start ANH. Reassurance can be given to families that medical evidence reports a peaceful death associated with cessation of ANH. Mouth care and hydration of lips and tongue with emollients can ease the feeling of dry mouth or chapped lips and allow the parents to continue the nurturing bond. Some children may find pleasure from tastes in their mouth; lollipops or candies can be used to facilitate this as well.

In some cases, the family distress about potential hunger or thirst can be significant, and it may be warranted to offer a trial of ANH and monitor closely for increased distressing symptoms. This shared decision-making process can relieve the parents' worry that they are not advocating enough for their child. If the trial is well tolerated, feeds or hydration can be given for a specified time frame with plans to discontinue if symptoms arise. Many children with complex medical needs have tube feeds as part of their normal medical care for years prior to their end-of-life phase. One could consider reducing the total volume of artificial feeds by 50–75% at end of life, which may be more acceptable to a family worried about their child experiencing hunger than stopping feeds altogether. Navigating the tension between benefits and burdens of these interventions can be challenging, but addressing the family concerns and finding a mutually agreed upon plan can facilitate discussions and ease tensions.

ANH are considered medical interventions and ethically can be withheld or withdrawn in cases of pediatric patients who are dying or severely incapacitated. The American Academy of Pediatrics (AAP) released guidelines in 2009 about withdrawing or withholding ANH in children. The report describes cases in which the burdens of ANH are greater than the benefits. Some situations in which the burdens of ANH could be greater than the benefits include persistent vegetative state, severe central nervous system anomalies, intestinal failure, severe congenital heart disease, end-stage malignancies, and actively dying patients. That is not to say that one must consider stopping or withholding ANH in this patient population but, rather, that attention should be paid to the burdens of medical interventions for high-risk patients. The AAP guidelines can help clarify the medical and ethical considerations in withdrawing and withholding ANH in pediatric patients. As with all decisions about medical interventions, discussion with caregivers should be done with empathy and attention to family perspectives on suffering and family values. ANH can have implications for many families' spiritual and cultural beliefs, so using professionals such as chaplains or community spiritual leaders to help navigate and explore family perspectives can help align the care of the patient to the family's values and goals.

The neonatal patient you were asked to see in the NICU is actively dying and already shows signs of hypoxia. As the infant's body continues to deteriorate, blood flow to her intestines will be shunted to her brain and heart, which will slow or stop digestion. Adding oral or gastric feeds at this time of active dying will likely add to the burden of suffering. Addressing the father's concerns about not starting feeds and exploring his worries will open the conversation to discuss this topic. Spend time intentionally listening to the father's concerns. Address the shutdown process of the body and the signs of cyanosis that you already are seeing in his daughter. Reassure him that he is doing everything he can for his daughter and that she is not feeling hungry or thirsty. You can touch on the fact that adding artificial hydration by way of intravenous fluids will likely worsen their daughter's respiratory distress. Invite the parents to perform oral care and apply emollients to their daughter's lips. Affirm the parent's love for their daughter and point out how beautifully they are taking care of her. If the infant's clinical status changes, you can readdress the issue of ANH at that time and consider a time trial of ANH or offer slow syringe feeds by mouth.

KEY POINTS TO REMEMBER

- Artificial nutrition and hydration are considered medical interventions. They can ethically be withdrawn or withheld from pediatric patients with severe disease burden in some situations.
- Providing nutrition and sustenance to children is a human instinct. Address this instinct and explore the emotional component of this topic.
- Engage in empathetic discussions with caregivers about burdens and benefits of ANH.
- Provide oral care and offer oral feeds or tastes if it is tolerated and provides comfort.
- Utilize spiritual leaders and chaplains to explore spiritual and cultural implications to ANH.

Further Reading

Casarett D, Kapo K, Caplan A. Appropriate use of artificial nutrition and hydration—Fundamental principles and recommendations. *N Engl J Med*. 2005;353(24):2607–2612.

Douglas S, Diekema DS, Botkin JR. Clinical report: Forgoing medically provided nutrition and hydration in children. The committee on bioethics. The American Academy of Pediatrics. *Pediatrics*. 2009;124(2w):813–822.

Rapoport A, Shaheed J, Newman C, Rugg M, Steele R. Parental perceptions of forgoing artificial nutrition and hydration during end-of-life care. *Pediatrics*. 2013;131(5):861–869.

Perinatal and Neonatal Care

27 Saying Hello and Goodbye

Lindsay B. Ragsdale

A 32-year-old pregnant female at 20 weeks of gestation is in the obstetrics (OB) clinic with her husband for prenatal ultrasound. They have been trying for a few years to get pregnant, and they were very excited to find out they were having their second child. The ultrasound took a long time to complete, and the sonographer had to bring in the physician to assist her with some images. The OB physician tells the couple that their infant has severe congenital heart disease and multiple significant anomalies with brain, lungs, and kidneys. They will pursue testing for a likely underlying genetic abnormality, but the prognosis is poor. The OB asks what their goals are for delivery and interventions at birth. They feel overwhelmed and unsure of what their goals are or even how to plan for delivery. They are referred to you to make a plan for delivery and care of the infant after birth.

What do you do now?

PERINATAL BIRTH PLANNING

Congenital anomalies found during prenatal ultrasound can be devastating for parents, and discussing options at delivery can be emotional and challenging. The Centers for Disease Control and Prevention reports that birth defects affect approximately 3% of all infants born in the United States each year, with variability in severity at birth depending on the defect. Mothers and parents can struggle with understanding the effects that the defects may have on quality of life and survivability. They may be asked their preference for cardiopulmonary resuscitation or surgeries after birth. Some of these decisions may affect the choice of pediatric center where the mother can deliver, requiring relocation prior to delivery. Parents can struggle with conversations about their infant's life and feel conflict with medical teams over goals of care. Many pediatric palliative teams offer prenatal counseling and birth planning to map out goals of care and a care plan at delivery.

Perinatal palliative care can include discussions of prenatal care, labor and delivery planning, care of the newborn after birth, postpartum care for the mother, memory-making, bereavement care, spiritual support, and/or postpartum depression screening and counseling. Often, this kind of planning takes place over multiple visits as trust and rapport build with the palliative care team. Prenatal care discussions can include conversations about whether to continue pregnancy to term, diagnostic testing, and the frequency of ultrasounds. Some families choose to continue pregnancy to term and want to hold their infant even if it will not live very long. No matter which choice a mother or couple makes, support for their goals should be given and their infant should be treated with respect and not just as a diagnosis.

Discussions about labor and delivery can include desire for standard vaginal delivery versus cesarean section and the mother's preference if she or her infant were in peril. These discussions should include OB providers, with attention to risks and benefits to mother and infant of each delivery option. Some centers can support home births in conjunction with a home care agency or hospice and take care of the infant after birth. Discussions regarding location of delivery should take place in conjunction with OB in order to ensure safe delivery for the mother and infant. Other details of labor and delivery to plan include which family members will be present in the delivery room, who will cut the umbilical cord, whether cord blood needs to be collected for testing, whether the placenta needs to be tested or preserved, and/or whether a neonatology or pediatric delivery team needs to be present for resuscitation.

The care of the newborn can vary greatly depending on the goals of care at birth. There are three main resuscitation plans at birth (although details can vary by case): comfort care, conditional resuscitation, and full resuscitative care. These care plans are on a spectrum between comfort only and full resuscitation, with conditional birth plans allowing some interventions but limiting others or changing courses during the resuscitation if the infant is unexpectedly better or worse than prenatally predicted. Comfort care at birth is described in detail, but keep in mind the details of a birth plan can be adapted for a family's particular spiritual or cultural beliefs or medical goals.

Comfort care at birth ensures that all aspects of care are aligned to alleviate and avoid pain. The infant is warmed and given closeness with family with swaddling or skin-to-skin contact depending on family desires. Medications are administered for pain or dyspnea, such as oral/buccal morphine or intranasal fentanyl with increasing frequency or dose as needed to control symptoms. Benzodiazepines can be given via oral/buccal or intranasal routes to control agitation or seizure activity. Discussions about utility versus burdens of blood tests, vaccines, state metabolic screens, eye ointment, and vitamin K injections after birth depend on the patient's prognosis. If the infant is expected to live only minutes or hours, these interventions may not be useful. Respiratory support at birth for comfort care should be discussed, as should the burdens versus benefits of supplemental oxygen and suctioning. Often, these interventions are not helpful to the infant at end of life and may make it difficult for family bonding. Nutrition for many infants with lethal anomalies may be difficult due to distress or inability to latch and suck; however, a mother may desire to attempt to feed with breast or bottle, and some families may choose to provide breast milk/formula or fluid by feeding tube. These feeding options should be discussed in detail, including the implications of feeding in the presence of respiratory distress or multiorgan dysfunction, which can worsen symptoms.

Allowing for parenting to occur during the postnatal period is crucial to provide an opportunity for bonding, cherishing time together, and memory-making. Teams can help facilitate memory-making activities with bathing, dressing, reading, singing, photos, keepsakes, mementos, birth celebrations, and/or dedications. Spiritual support from a local spiritual leader or hospital chaplain can be very helpful for some families; many pediatric palliative programs have palliative chaplains embedded in their teams who can provide spiritual support. Allowing time and space for families to be with their infant in the location of birth can help facilitate these important bonding experiences.

Home care may be needed if the infant survives longer than expected and the mother is ready for discharge from the hospital. Home hospice teams can continue comfort care at home and provide on-call symptom support for the infant. The hospice team can continue the interdisciplinary care of the entire family and provide bereavement support if the infant dies at home. Depending on how long the infant is expected to survive, a primary care physician may need to be identified in order to provide routine pediatric care. If the prognosis is longer than a few days' survival, you can consider giving the infant a vitamin K injection to prevent potential hemorrhagic disease of the newborn after discharge. The low risk of this more rare neonatal complication should be balanced with the invasiveness of the injection.

Postmortem care of the infant can include discussions of genetic testing or specimen collection, autopsy, and funeral home transitions and planning. Mothers may benefit from a lactation consultant visit, if available, or education about the lactation process after the loss of an infant. After discharge from the hospital, bereavement follow-up and coordination with grief counseling resources can be helpful for grieving parents and provide ongoing support as their grief changes over time.

Perinatal birth planning can help facilitate discussions about goals of care and ensure treatment teams understand the situation at delivery. Reflecting back to the initial case of the parents with an infant with prenatal diagnosis of multiple congenital anomalies, initial discussions should focus on understanding the diagnosis and identifying central goals of care. Future discussions can expand the conversation to include details of labor and delivery and care of the infant. All of these care discussions should include respect for parent choices, providing psychosocial and spiritual support, honoring the life of the infant, and creating an opportunity for parenting and incorporation into the family.

KEY POINTS TO REMEMBER

- Provide nonjudgmental care with respect for parent preferences.
- Identify central goals of care and family values.
- Create birth plan that reflects the parents' choices.
- There are three main birth plans: comfort care, conditional resuscitation, and full resuscitation.
- For the comfort care birth plan, ensure all aspects of care align with the comfort of the infant and bonding with family.
- Honor the importance of the life of the infant.
- Provide psychosocial and spiritual support for grief.

Further Reading

Centers for Disease Control and Prevention. Update on overall prevalence of major birth defects—Atlanta, Georgia, 1978–2005. *MMWR Morbid Mortal Wkly Rep.* 2008;57(1):1–5. Retrieved from https://www.cdc.gov/mmwr/preview/mmwrhtml/mm5701a2.htm

Denney-Koelsch E, et al. A survey of perinatal palliative care programs in the United States: Structure, processes, and outcomes. *J Palliat Med.* 2016;19(10):1080–1086.

English NK, Hessler KL. Prenatal birth planning for families of the imperiled newborn. *J Obstet Gynecol Neonatal Nurs.* 2013;42:390–399.

Guon J, Wilfond BS, Farlow B, Brazg T, Janvier A. Our children are not a diagnosis: The experience of parents who continue their pregnancy after a prenatal diagnosis of trisomy 13 or 18. *Am J Med Genet.* 2014;164(Part A):308–318.

28 I Feel My Baby Moving; How Is She Incompatible with Life?

Lindsay B. Ragsdale

You are asked to see a 29-year-old first-time mother who is 30 weeks pregnant. On ultrasound, the fetus is lagging 4 weeks behind in growth and has clenched hands and signs of duodenal atresia. The mother has been informed of the high suspicion of trisomy 18 by her family obstetrician (OB) and was told that her baby was "incompatible with life." She was advised not to bring a car seat to her delivery because her baby was not going to survive long enough to go home with her. She is heartbroken and feels her baby moving inside of her, which gives her hope that her daughter may beat the odds. She joined an online community for parents of children with trisomy 18 and was shocked to learn that some children can live years. She does not want her daughter to suffer, but she does not want to "give up" on her either. She asks your advice on how to care for her daughter after birth and what she can anticipate regarding survival and quality of life.

What do you do now?

FETAL DIAGNOSIS OF TRISOMY 13 AND 18

Trisomy 13 and 18, the presence of an extra chromosome 13 or 18, respectively, have historically been categorized as "lethal" anomalies, with many neonates dying quickly after birth. Trisomy 13 and 18 are associated with severe neurodevelopmental impairment, congenital heart disease, intestinal obstructions/malformations, brain anomalies, central apnea, musculoskeletal deformities, cleft lip and palate, neural tube defects, hearing loss, feeding difficulties, growth restriction, and eye anomalies. Many patients with trisomy 13 or 18 will have a combination of these conditions, and many require surgical interventions for continued survival. The developmental delay associated with these syndromes is usually significant, and most affected individuals have little or no speech development or ambulation. Due to improved and more widespread prenatal testing, parents are finding out sooner during pregnancy about the diagnosis. The early diagnosis creates an opportunity to begin an honest conversation about potential outcomes in order to help families readjust to their new reality and start to plan for the future.

After receiving the prenatal diagnosis of trisomy 13 or 18, many parents choose not to continue the pregnancy. Some parents who have chosen to continue the pregnancy have been told their infant is "incompatible with life." Historical data supports the conclusion that these infants died quickly after birth, with 50% dying within the first week of life. Recent data show that these infants are being offered surgical interventions such as cardiac surgeries, shunts, feeding tubes, and abdominal surgeries, and as a result many children are living longer. Data suggest that infants with trisomy 13 and 18 are still at risk for death in the first month of life; however, there appears to be a subset of infants who can survive longer with medical support and surgery. For infants with trisomy 13 or 18 who survive until 6 months of age, the chances of longer term survival increase greatly. Five-year survival is estimated in some studies as 10% for trisomy 13 and 12% for trisomy 18. Early gestational age at birth is an independent risk factor for increased mortality in both trisomy 13 and trisomy 18. These new data reflect a change in survival compared to previously reported data. The change in survival may reflect a shift in thought about trisomy 13 and 18 and an increased willingness for some centers to offer surgeries and more aggressive medical interventions for this population.

Survival is not the only outcome that is meaningful. Quality of life for these infants plays an important role in navigating their care plan long term. Little has been published on the quality of life of long-term survivors, and attention needs to be given to managing symptoms and relieving suffering. Intermittent assessment of suffering and readdressing family goals and values over time can ensure continued alignment of medical care. Creating opportunities to explore the family's experience with their child's illness and how the family is coping with the experience can help address gaps and give anticipatory guidance. The conversation can start prenatally to begin to prepare a family for the potential health challenges and high risk of early death. As difficult as these conversations can be, parents appreciate honest and empathetic conversations and want providers to address their hopes and fears. Parents of children with trisomy 13 and 18 have expressed the concern that some medical providers do not treat their unborn child as a person or as important. Medical providers should approach these conversations with curiosity about the family's journey and give respect to their child as an important part of their family.

Perinatal birth planning can help identify the family's central goals and values, and this process can help guide resuscitation efforts and begin the discussion of the boundaries of potential medical interventions. Birth planning can be helpful for the parents to wrestle with these difficult decisions before they are in a crisis moment at birth. Delivery and resuscitative interventions can be mapped out prior to delivery and shared with obstetric and neonatal providers. Throughout the pregnancy and after birth, emotional and spiritual support should be offered for the parents and siblings. Many parents grieve the loss of the healthy infant they might have been expecting and struggle with the new challenges that face their child and their family. Normalizing this experience can help relieve the isolation that can occur during this process. Some centers have layered in memory-making during pregnancy, including fetal heartbeat recording, heartbeat recording incorporated into a chosen song, framed ultrasound pictures, and prenatal pictures. These activities emphasize the importance of the infant in their family structure and help the family focus on enjoying each moment with their infant prenatally. Many parents have described being given bad news at each prenatal clinic appointment; these activities can counter that negativity and serve as a source of joy and bonding for parents, while clinicians can remain honest regarding prognosis following birth. Collaboration with OB and ultrasound professionals can help facilitate these activities prior to birth.

In the neonatal period, the health challenges to successful discharge home can include central apnea, cardiac dysfunction, and feeding difficulty. Exploring family goals and matching the goals with potential medical interventions can help set realistic expectations. Community resources such as home palliative and hospice teams can help patients with symptom management and provide ongoing support for the family. Long-term survivors with trisomy 13 and 18 usually require ongoing medical support and are at risk for repeated inpatient admissions. Palliative teams can join with families to advocate for medical needs as their children with trisomy 13 and 18 change over time.

The pregnant mother you were asked to see is asking for guidance relating to prognosis and expectations for her daughter. You sit down with her to hear what her pregnancy journey has been like for her. You explore her feelings of grief for the perfect baby she was anticipating and the fears of what her daughter might experience after birth. She wants to know all of the details of medical care and prognosis that you are willing to share. You take your time to explain about trisomy 18 and the changing data concerning prognosis and mortality. You talk about the most common medical conditions that infants with trisomy 18 can face and how family values factor into decision-making concerning the boundaries of medical interventions. After exploring her ideas of good quality of life, together you develop a plan for her infant to have a full resuscitation at birth and for her to go to the neonatal intensive care unit (NICU). You discuss with the mother the evaluation that her daughter will undergo and the challenges that her daughter will have regarding independent breathing and feeding. The mother will be scheduled with pediatric surgery to discuss duodenal atresia repair and surgical expectations. She is hopeful that her daughter will be a long-term survivor but wants to be realistic about the risk of death. You discuss with her plans if her daughter is born with more severe anomalies than anticipated. She would want honest communication and would decide at that point to focus on her daughter's comfort and try to take her home without painful procedures. She wants to have her daughter baptized by her local pastor after delivery. She is thankful for your candor and for allowing her to explore her hopes and fears with you. You communicate your conversation to her OB and the NICU team.

> **KEY POINTS TO REMEMBER**
>
> - Trisomy 13 and 18 are diagnoses no longer thought of as "incompatible with life." Medical care and surgeries can be offered and should align with family goals.
> - Infants with trisomy 13 and 18 can have a significant burden of illness, including cardiac, gastrointestinal, neurologic, and developmental.
> - Fifty percent of infants with trisomy 13 and 18 die before 1 week of life.
> - Long-term survival rates of affected infants are higher after 6 months of life, and some patients can live for years.
> - Quality of life can be significantly impacted by multiorgan involvement. Ongoing assessments should address suffering and family values.

Further Reading

Côté-Arsenault D, Denney-Koelsch E. "My baby is a person": Parents' experiences with life-threatening fetal diagnosis. *J Palliat Med.* 2011;14(12):1302–1308.

Jenkins KJ, Roberts AE. Trisomy 13 and 18: Cardiac surgery makes sense if it is part of a comprehensive care strategy. *Pediatrics.* 2017;140(5):e20172809.

Kosiv KA, Gossett JM, Bai S, Collins RT. Congenital heart surgery on in-hospital mortality in trisomy 13 and 18. *Pediatrics.* 2017;140(5):e20170772.

Nelson KE, Rosella LC, Mahant S, Guttmann A. Survival and surgical interventions for children with trisomy 13 and 18. *JAMA.* 2016;316(4):420–428.

29 A Moment Becomes a Memory

Lindsay B. Ragsdale

You are asked to come to the labor and delivery ward urgently to see an infant who was just born precipitously. The mother had no prenatal care because she did not know she was pregnant. The newborn has an absence of the top of the skull and forehead, and a small amount of brain tissue is visible through a thin membrane covering the top of the head. The newborn's eyes are proptotic bilaterally. The newborn is gasping intermittently and has a heart rate less than 60 beats per minute. The infant is nonresponsive, and there is little or no movement of his extremities. The mother is in shock that she was pregnant and is having difficulty looking at her infant. The obstetric (OB) nurses are asking what they should do to help the infant and the mother.

What do you do now?

ANENCEPHALY AND OTHER BRAIN REDUCTION ABNORMALITIES

Anencephaly, with an incidence of 1 in 1,000–2,000 births, is a fatal congenital malformation of the brain in which little or no brain is present at birth. Anencephaly is a neural tube defect that results from incomplete fusion of the neural tube during early embryogenesis. As the embryo grows, the open brain tissue is directly exposed to amniotic fluid, which causes destruction of the neural tissue. The small amount of remaining brain tissue, only small remnants of cerebellum and brain stem, is covered by a thin membrane. Neonates with anencephaly typically have no scalp or skull and little or no forehead and prominent eyes as seen in Figure 29.1. The etiology of anencephaly is thought to be due to maternal folate deficiency, genetic abnormalities, or environmental/toxin exposures. The pregnancy has a high risk of intrauterine fetal demise and stillbirth. If the infant is born alive, the condition is usually fatal within hours to days. There have been a few case reports worldwide of infants with anencephaly living for months or years; however, these are rare and their diagnosis of classic anencephaly has been

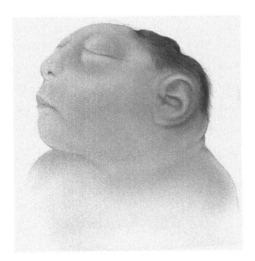

FIGURE 29.1 Neonate with anencephaly.

Source: Image courtesy of the Centers for Disease Control and Prevention, National Center on Birth Defects and Developmental Disabilities.

controversial. There are no medical interventions to treat the anencephaly, but layering in symptom management and support for family is crucial.

Pregnant mothers are routinely offered pregnancy termination, where legally available, after the diagnosis of anencephaly is discovered, and many families choose this option. However, some families choose to continue the pregnancy until birth. Early conversations about what to expect of pregnancy, labor, and time with the infant are important to modulate expectations and identify family goals. Parents should be advised about the classic appearance of anencephaly and what they can expect. Some families have appreciated gentle discussions about the exposed brain and options for covering the top of the head if they desire with petroleum-coated gauze (to prevent tissues adhering) and a bonnet or hat with ties under the chin. Some families have asked about what their infant may feel or be able to sense after birth. Although there is no evidence regarding the extent of sensorium of infants with anencephaly, some have been able to breathe on their own for a period of time, cry, feed, react to stimulation, and blink; however, higher level consciousness is not thought to be present. Parents should be supported as they give love and tenderness to their infant with the goal of savoring each moment with the infant. Many parents who continue the pregnancy have reported goals to spend time with their infant, share love, meet siblings and family members, take family photos, participate in spiritual rituals, and have an opportunity to parent their infant. These goals can be supported with preparation of staff and involvement of the perinatal palliative care team or other specialized team sensitive to these needs. Parents should be given the opportunity to explore their wishes and to map out their desires for their baby and family at birth. A birth plan can aid in communication of family goals to the OB and neonatal services.

Neonates who are born alive with anencephaly may have symptoms of respiratory distress at birth. First-line treatment of respiratory distress in neonates is opioids, which can be administered via oral, intranasal, or sublingual routes. Many centers use sublingual morphine 0.1–0.2 mg/kg every 30 minutes as needed for respiratory distress and have these doses available prior to delivery to avoid a gap in time of availability. Reassurance to family about changes they are witnessing as the infant declines can help provide context and relieve parental concerns. Use of supplemental oxygen will not likely be helpful for symptom management and may prolong suffering, but these decisions should align with family goals. Focus on comfort at birth should help guide other medical care, including avoiding painful procedures or injections.

Some families have expressed the need that their infant's life and death be meaningful, and they want the ability to help others. In the 1990s, some centers in the United States began to consider infants with anencephaly as potential organ donor candidates. There is a very long waiting list for organ recipients, and many die waiting for organs because the demand has outstripped the supply of organs. Considering anencephalic infants as organ donation candidates allows for the potential to meet the need of the donor family of a meaningful legacy and meet the need of the recipient for organs and prolonged life. Some organ procurement organizations have considered this population for tissue donation (heart valves and corneas) after death, but these infants are not routinely considered candidates for organ donation for transplant outside of research protocols at this time.

Other congenital brain reduction abnormalities, such as hydranencephaly, congenital hydrocephalus, holoprosencephaly, schizencephaly, and lissencephaly, can be due to malformations or disruptions during embryogenesis. They can have a spectrum of severity and survival. Infants affected by these abnormalities can have a significant disease burden and symptoms affecting quality of life. Involvement of a palliative program early in the infant's life can help the family identify goals and readjust medical care that aligns with their goals as the infant ages. Many infants with brain abnormalities, especially those with severe pathology, require medications, medical technologies, and therapies. These patients are at higher risk for acute events, recurrent admissions, and quality of life challenges. Palliative programs can attend to these challenges and help families navigate medical care along the disease trajectory.

The neonatal case you are asked to see in labor and delivery has clinical features consistent with anencephaly. You have examined the infant gently and observed the absence of skull bones and scalp. You see a thin membrane over small remnants of brain tissue at the base of the skull. The infant's eyes are prominent with little eye movement. The infant has only subtle movement of extremities, although she has significant respiratory distress with intermittent gasping. You introduce yourself to the mother and ask her what she knows about her baby so far and how much detail she would like to know about her baby. She has calmed from the initial shock and wants to know more details about her baby. You describe your exam, diagnosis of anencephaly, and the grave prognosis. You talk about focusing on the comfort of her daughter and that you want to give medications in her daughter's mouth to help her shortness of breath. You acknowledge how difficult it must be to find out about pregnancy and anencephaly at the same time. You talk about wanting to ensure comfort and discuss with the mother about being with her baby. You ask about her feelings seeing her daughter's head, and she admits that seeing the top of the head was traumatic for her. You suggest adding a petroleum gauze cover and a bonnet to cover the exposed head, dressing her in an outfit, and wrapping her in a warm blanket. The mother feels comfortable with this plan and is excited to see her daughter in a newborn outfit because she did not have anything prepared and was feeling guilty. After you treat the infant's respiratory distress and put her in an outfit, you bring her to her mother. She is tearful and excited to see her daughter. She is able to take pictures with her, sing and read baby books to her. Your team records the infant's heartbeat and makes a memory album with her hand- and footprints. Her daughter dies 3 hours later. The mother is appreciative of the time she had with her daughter and the opportunity to bond with her. You discuss grief counseling and ensure follow-up for her after discharge from the hospital.

KEY POINTS TO REMEMBER

- Anencephaly is a lethal neural tube defect with typical absence of skull and scalp with exposed brain remnants and brain stem.
- Some parents choose to continue the pregnancy; neonates with anencephaly can be born alive and live hours to days.
- Symptom management medications may be needed for respiratory distress at birth for neonates with anencephaly.
- Supporting parental bond and family goals should be the focus at birth.
- Other brain abnormalities can range in severity and survival; palliative programs can attend to quality of life and disease burdens.

Further Reading

Centers for Disease Control and Prevention. Facts about anencephaly. Retrieved from
https://www.cdc.gov/ncbddd/birthdefects/anencephaly.html

Côté-Arsenault D, Denney-Koelsch E. "Have no regrets": Parents' experiences and
developmental tasks in pregnancy with a lethal fetal diagnosis. *Social Sci Med.*
2016;154:100–109.

Jaquier M, Klein A, Boltshauser E. Spontaneous pregnancy outcome after prenatal
diagnosis of anencephaly. *BJOG.* 2006;113(8): 951–953.

Obeidi N, Russell N, Higgins JR, O'Donoghue K. The natural history of anencephaly.
Prenat Diagn. 2010;30(4):357–360.

O'Connell O, Meaney S, O'Donoghue K. Anencephaly—The maternal experience
of continuing with the pregnancy: Incompatible with life but not with love.
Midwifery. 2019;71:12–18.

30 Tiny Fingers, Tiny Toes

Lindsay B. Ragsdale

You are consulted on a premature newborn in the neonatal intensive care unit (NICU) who was born this morning at 23.1 weeks of gestation due to premature rupture of membranes at 16 weeks with premature labor since yesterday. The neonate weighs 425 g, is on high-frequency ventilation, requires two medications for blood pressure support, and has had a drop in hematocrit since this morning concerning for an intraventricular hemorrhage. The mother is still admitted to the obstetrics service and is recovering from delivery. You examine the infant and then go to the mother's room to find out how they are coping with the NICU admission. When you walk into her room, there are 12 other family members in the room with her, including the father, and they are all crying. You introduce yourself and discuss how you can give support long term in the NICU and beyond. The mother is crying and says she does not think she will need your services because her baby will likely die today anyway.

What do you do now?

PREMATURITY AND ROCKY NEONATAL COURSE

Preterm birth is defined as birth prior to 37 weeks of gestation, with further classification into moderate or late preterm (32–37 weeks), very preterm (28–32 weeks), and extremely preterm (less than 28 weeks). Sequelae of prematurity increase in incidence and severity at earlier gestations, with neurodevelopmental disabilities almost a certainty among survivors at 22 weeks. Based on the most recent US data from the National Institute of Child Health and Human Development: Neonatal Research Network and Pedatrix studies, the chances of survival are less than 10% at 22 weeks, 40–50% at 23 weeks, 60–70% at 24 weeks, and 75–78% at 25 weeks. Survival rates of extremely premature neonates have been increasing during the past 10 years, but survival alone is the not the only important outcome. The long-term impact of neurocognitive and physical disabilities can be significant for patients and their families, highlighting the importance of honest conversations about quality of life and family goals. Many pediatric palliative teams meet premature neonates early in the NICU course to help support families and walk this unpredictable journey with them. Palliative team involvement can help not only if the neonate succumbs to prematurity-related diseases but also because of the long-term implications to quality of life, psychosocial stress, sibling support, resource needs, risk for readmissions, and technology dependence.

The NICU course for a premature neonate has been described by many parents as a rollercoaster with different phases, depending on the clinical course: the crisis admission phase, the middle marathon phase, and the discharge phase. The first phase of NICU admission can be a shock to parents who were not anticipating early delivery. The first few days can be an overwhelming experience, and parents may have difficulty grasping the severity or long-term implications of their infant being born early. Parents have described grieving the loss of the "normal" pregnancy and losing the ability to enjoy the preparation phase of taking home a healthy newborn. Mothers have shared the experience of feeling phantom baby movements inside of them only to remember they have already delivered, or sadness of never even feeling their baby move if delivery is extremely premature. Parents have expressed the difficulty bonding with a very small infant who is connected to machines, and they often do not have the opportunity to hold the infant at the beginning. These delayed bonding moments can arrest the development of parental bonding and make it challenging for parents at first. Guidance and reassurance can help parents form a bond in a different way than they had expected through involvement in daily care such as mouth care, changing diapers, reading, and gentle touching. Child life specialists can help with these bonding activities and can involve siblings if the NICU protocol allows. Parents with infants in the NICU are at higher risk for depression, anxiety, and trauma symptoms, and mothers are particularly at higher risk for postpartum depression. NICUs should have increased sensitivity to this increased risk and have supports in place to screen and refer parents in need of support. Many palliative teams have mental health professionals available, as well, for support of parents in the NICU.

The second phase of many NICU admissions is the middle marathon phase, in which the neonate has survived past the initial crisis of admission and now is working on lung development and growth, which can often take months. The parents have usually worked through the shock of prematurity and have grown accustomed to the NICU environment and equipment. Many parents have created a schedule of visitation and are involved in care of the infant. This phase can be difficult for parents to maintain their employment, pay their bills, and plan for taking family leave, and they may feel despondent about the length of stay. Acknowledgment of these challenges can help parents not feel alone in the process, and connecting them to psychosocial resources can ease the financial and social impacts of prolonged NICU stay. Siblings can have difficulty adjusting to a prolonged disruption in their family rhythms. Families can help siblings adjust to the "new normal" and to still feel important and loved. Child life services in many centers can work with children to understand their sibling's illness and participate in coping and bonding activities.

Medical sequelae such as intraventricular hemorrhage (IVH), bronchopulmonary dysplasia (BPD), feeding difficulties, and pulmonary hypertension can be discovered during the middle marathon phase. These diagnoses can change the potential outcomes for patients and can drastically change the care they require at home. Infants with severe BPD and feeding difficulties may require a tracheostomy, home ventilator, or gastric tube. These technologies may be new to parents, and the benefits/burdens of care should be explored with them prior to surgery. Parents may need to readjust their expectations of what they thought their child's life was going to be like in the future, either for the next few years or over their child's lifetime. The realization of potential prognosis can cause sadness and grief for families. Teams should acknowledge this grief, explore the family's ideas of good quality of life, and discuss options. Some parents may want to change goals if the prognosis is grave and the anticipated quality of life is not what they wanted for their child.

The final phase of a NICU admission is the discharge phase, in which care is transitioned to home with supporting technology as needed. Parents may have mixed emotions about taking their child home—excitement for finally getting home and also fear about medical care being solely their responsibility. Teams should allow space for both of these emotions and to ensure a discharge plan that addresses caregiver concerns. The discharge planning process can vary in length and intensity, and it may require parents to stay at the hospital to demonstrate competency. Some parents may have become close with staff members in the hospital and may have to grapple with the "loss" of their medical teams. Connecting parents with new supports at home and in the community may help transition the support they were receiving in the hospital. Many families retain long-term connections with the NICU and return for "NICU graduate" activities.

Some former premature infants have ongoing medical needs and may require readmissions to the hospital during illnesses. These infants may be admitted to a new unit in which their medical history is not known as intimately as it was known in the NICU, and caregivers may need to advocate for their child in a way they did not need to during the neonatal period. The parent transitions their role to the "expert" on their child and may need to readjust to a new unit or medical team. The parent may experience significant personal growth during this time, which can be unexpected but also empowering. Many inpatient palliative care teams can be a source of continuity for parents from the NICU to other inpatient units. Palliative teams can provide medical context to the new pediatric teams and can also help parents care for their child over time with attention to family goals and quality of life.

The case that you were asked to see is a 23-week premature neonate with critical medical issues and concerns for survival. You are talking with the mother and her family about their goals and concerns. The mother is tearful and concerned that her baby is going to die, and she desperately wants him to survive. You ask her to talk more about this worry and what she has been told about her son's condition. She says that the NICU team explained to her that due to her son's gestational age, he is at risk for complications of prematurity, even death. She said that after she heard the word "death," she did not register anything else that they said. She explains that she is a special education teacher and takes care of neurodevelopmentally impaired children and believes that they have a good quality of life. She wants to pursue every avenue to ensure her son has a chance to survive. You invite the NICU team back to the bedside to continue the conversation with the mother about expected survival and outcomes. The mother hears from the NICU team that her son has been slowly improving today with the need for only one medication for blood pressure support and has a grade III IVH on head ultrasound. They acknowledge the risks for her son's survival and outcome but assure her that they will do everything medically they can that will help him. During the next few weeks, the baby improves, and you are able to establish good rapport with the family. You see him throughout his NICU admission and also follow him for several years during repeat admissions to the pediatric ICU. He has moderate to severe developmental delay and technology dependence. His mother is so happy to spend each day with him and is appreciative of the care he has received. He is able to be in her special education class at school, and she believes that his quality of life is great.

KEY POINTS TO REMEMBER

- Preterm birth includes moderate or late preterm (32–37 weeks), very preterm (28–32 weeks), and extremely preterm (less than 28 weeks).
- Neurodevelopmental disabilities increase in incidence and severity with earlier gestational age at birth.
- NICU admissions can have phases: the crisis admission phase, the middle marathon phase, and the discharge phase. These phases can be challenging for parents, and support should be extended to address concerns and discuss expectations.

- Parents and families can experience significant stress during a NICU admission and are high risk for mental health issues.
- Premature infants are at higher risk for neurodevelopmental and physical challenges that can impact their quality of life.

Further Reading

Ecker JL, Mercer BM, Blackwell SC, et al. Periviable birth: Interim update. *Am J Obstet Gynecol.* 2016;215(2):B2–B12.

Luu TM, Rehman Mian MO, Nuyt AM. Long-term impact of preterm birth: Neurodevelopmental and physical health outcomes. *Clin Perinatol.* 2017;44(2):305–314.

National Institute of Child Health and Human Development, Neonatal Research Network. Retrieved from https://neonatal.rti.org

Obeidat HM, Bond E, Callister L. The parental experience of having an infant in the newborn intensive care unit. *J Perinatal Educ.* 2009;18(3):23–29.

Patel RM, Rysavy MA, Bell EF, Tyson JE. Survival of infants born at periviable gestational ages. *Clin Perinatol.* 2017;44(2):287–303.

Younge N, Goldstein RF, Bann CM, et al. Survival and neurodevelopmental outcomes among periviable infants. *N Engl J Med.* 2017;376(7):617–628.

Adolescent and Young Adult Care

31   A Case of Refusing to Agree

Kelstan Ellis and Jennifer Linebarger

You are seeing a 16-year-old female who recently moved to the area. A year ago, she was diagnosed with medulloblastoma and underwent gross total resection. Her oncologist recommended radiation followed by chemotherapy that offered a 5-year event-free survival of 85%. After discussions, she underwent radiation therapy and had a variety of expected but bothersome side effects, including nausea, throat irritation, and cognitive difficulties (short-term memory loss). The patient and family had delayed follow-up for chemotherapy because of the move to your area.

During your first visit, the patient reports that she does not want to undergo chemotherapy, stating "it is toxic to my body," and expresses interest in alternative therapies. Based on limited data, foregoing timely chemotherapy places the patient's expected 5-year event-free survival at approximately 50%. Her parents want to be supportive of their daughter but remain interested in initiating chemotherapy.

What do you do now?

DEFINE ASSENT AND CONSENT

In the medical setting, a competent adult must give informed consent for medical interventions such as chemotherapy. Such a framework is designed to respect a person's autonomy, often referred to as "respect of persons." Consent requires the legal ability to enter into contract with adequate knowledge and information. As such, within pediatric medicine, consent is given by the legal guardian (typically the parents). Children, particularly adolescents, are involved in decisions regarding medical decision-making by offering assent. Assent refers to the child's agreement to medical treatments in circumstances in which they are not legally authorized to give consent. The legal authorization is often based on age, and the age limits for consent vary widely across nations and states and may depend on the treatment in question (e.g., treatment of sexually transmitted infections).

Assent should be an interactive and ongoing process between the clinician and the pediatric patient. In ideal circumstances, patient assent would be obtained prior to treatment initiation, even when it is assumed legal guardians are making decisions and offering consent in the patient's best interest. It is imperative to seek balance in prioritizing assent and consent in order to both protect children's interests when they are not fully able to do so themselves and respect their autonomy when they can exercise it.

Two additional terms that frequently appear in discussions of consent and assent are capacity and competence. Capacity is a developmental term referring to differing levels of abilities to synthesize information. Prior personal experiences with decision-making can contribute to these abilities, as can the specifics of disease processes. Competence is a legal term regarding the degree of capacity sufficient to make a decision. It is important to note that this is not the same as agreeing with the medical team. Capacity can be determined by a clinician or researcher, whereas a judge or other legal entity may be required to determine competence. Common components of capacity include the ability to understand the information provided, make comparisons of the options (reasoning skills), infer consequences or appreciate the effect of the information, and express a choice. As such, capacity can change over time. Capacity can also be decision specific, meaning an individual may have capacity to make some choices, such as determining who they would like to help them make medical decisions, but lack capacity for more complex decisions such as forgoing a life-sustaining treatment.

ASSESS

When determining the capacity to provide consent or assent, providers should take into account age, maturity (including disease experience), psychological state of the individual, as well as the type of decision and the level of risk:benefit the decision entails. For example, assent is not sought prior to administration of vaccines to an infant because the patient lacks the developmental capacity to understand the medical intervention and the benefits of vaccination. Older children may be able to participate in the decision-making processes even if they are not mature enough to provide true assent—for example, a school-age child deciding in which arm to receive a vaccine.

The American Academy of Pediatrics (AAP) recommends the following steps for soliciting a child's assent:

- Help the patient achieve awareness of his or her condition.
- Tell the patient what to expect regarding diagnosis and treatment.
- Assess the patient's understanding.
- Assess for factors influencing the patient response.
- Solicit the patient's willingness to accept care.

Similarly, the AAP has recommendations on the components of informed consent:

- Provision of information, including explanation (in understandable language) of the diagnosis, proposed interventions, probability of success, risks and benefits, and alternatives to treatment (including the option not to treat)
- Assessment of the understanding of information provided
- Assessment of the decision-maker's capacity to provide consent
- Assurance, when possible, that the decision-maker is free to choose among medical options without manipulation or coercion from the medical team

For both assent and consent, it is important to provide thorough and accurate information and strive to facilitate open and honest communication between all parties involved.

WHEN THERE IS DISAGREEMENT

Many parents believe that the decisions concerning their child's life are theirs to make, regardless of the child's awareness or capacity. The desire to provide consent without involving the child is often a combination of exercising the traditional role of a parent and a desire to do what the parents believe is in the child's best interest. Sometimes parents or caregivers do not believe their child is capable of understanding the complexities of decision-making, others wish to spare their child from what can be emotional and difficult discussions, and still others may not be aware that it is acceptable to include their children in the decision-making process. When a guardian voices concern about "truth telling," it warrants further conversation. Such concerns may be influenced by previous experiences, cultural and religious influences, family traditions, and many more factors.

Most children do not expect to make decisions on their own; rather, they want to be involved in the process and have their opinions respected. This can be called "collaborative paternalism," in which children are given the opportunity to express their thoughts, concerns, and preferences with the expectation that the ultimate decision will be made by parents in concert with the medical team. As with all situations involving assent and consent, such collaborative paternalism should be considered in the context of a patient's age, development, and maturity level.

As children progress into adolescence, it is developmentally expected that there will be an increase in their autonomy. Some adolescents will be ready to take on more ownership, whereas others will shy away from such responsibilities. Parents and providers can help adolescents transition to become autonomous adults by fostering open communication, continually assessing their desire to be involved, and demonstrating respect for the adolescent's decisions and choices, when appropriate.

In circumstances in which a pediatric patient refuses to provide assent, how to continue with the treatment plan should be considered carefully. Proceeding without assent may negatively impact the patient–physician relationship. The motivation for refusal should be assessed. Frequently, refusal stems from a lack of sufficient understanding, underlying fear, and/or additional social considerations. There are helpful resources that can serve as guides to assist clinicians and researchers when seeking assent or when there is discord within the patient–parent–practitioner triad.

The following is a summary of relevant considerations from the American Medical Association's (AMA) Code of Medical Ethics:

- Involve patients in decision-making at a developmentally appropriate level.
- Include discussion of risks, benefits, alternatives, and prognosis in treatment recommendations.
- In patients capable of assent, truthfully explain the diagnosis and treatment plan with consideration of cognitive and emotional maturity.
- Provide a supportive environment and facilitate open communication.
- Recognize that disclosing certain health conditions may have unexpected consequences and disrupt relationships within the family.
- Involve patients, as appropriate based on their ability to understand and desire to participate, in decisions regarding life-sustaining interventions. Ensure patient and caregiver understanding of these interventions, and define goals and timelines to assess clinical effectiveness.
- If it is unclear whether a specific intervention promotes the patient's best interest, respect the decisions of the patients and parents/guardians.

The AMA suggests that in certain circumstances, consultation with the institution's ethics committee and involvement of risk management or outside regulatory entities may be necessary to resolve disagreements. In its conclusion, the AMA states that physicians should "provide compassionate and humane care to all pediatric patients, including patients who forgo or discontinue life-sustaining interventions."

In health care, clinicians strive to inform their patients to the best of their abilities and work with patients to formulate plans of care that are consistent with sound medical judgment and patients' goals. These efforts can be complicated in the pediatric population, in which patients are typically unable to provide consent. However, pediatric patients should be involved in medical decision-making to a level that is developmentally appropriate and desired by each individual. Circumstances in which patients or parents do not provide assent or consent, respectively, can be emotionally and clinically difficult for providers but should not be viewed as insurmountable. By understanding the components of assent and consent as well as the limits of each, practitioners can navigate these complicated scenarios while maintaining their clinical integrity and working toward the best interest of the patient.

The 16-year-old in our case very much wanted to be involved in decision-making about her cancer treatment. She had undergone surgery and radiation but did not want to undergo chemotherapy. She clearly articulated the risks of undergoing treatment and of declining further treatment. The medical team and her parents took her concerns seriously and further explored her worries about the chemotherapy and found them to be possible and not preventable. The medical team also could not clearly define "timely" delivery of chemotherapy and thought it possible that the treatment may not be as beneficial as initially described. Together, the patient, parents, and physician agreed that the benefits of "forcing" chemotherapy were not worth the harm to the patient's autonomy, relationship with her parents, and trust in the medical system.

KEY POINTS TO REMEMBER

- Assent is provided by the child, where consent is obtained from the parent/legal guardian when the child is not legally able to provide consent due to age.
- Assent should be an interactive and ongoing discussion that is tailored to the child's age, developmental status, and maturity level.
- When differences between children's and parents' desires are present, it is important to elicit motivation from all parties

involved, foster open communication, and seek to balance the best interest of the patient.

- If there is a reversible life-threatening condition and the patient or parents/guardians are refusing treatment, consider involving the institution's ethics committee.

Further Reading

American Medical Association. Pediatric decision making. In AMA Principles of Medical Ethics: IV, VIII. Retrieved from https://www.ama-assn.org/delivering-care/ethics/pediatric-decision-making

Bluebond-Langer M, Belasco JB, Wander MD. "I want to live, until I don't want to live anymore": Involving children with life-threatening and life-shortening illnesses in decision making about care and treatment. *Nurs Clin North Am.* 2010;45(3):329–343.

Katz AL, Webb SA; American Academy of Pediatrics Committee on Bioethics. Informed consent in decision-making in pediatric practice. *Pediatrics.* 2016;138(2):20161485.

McCabe MA. Involving children and adolescents in medical decision making: Developmental and clinical considerations. *J Pediatr Psychol.* 1996;21(4):505–516.

Rosenberg AR, Starks H, Unguru Y, Feudtner C, Diekema D. Truth telling in the setting of cultural differences and incurable pediatric illness. *JAMA Pediatr.* 2017;171(11):1113–1119.

Sisk BA, DuBois J, Kodish E, Wolfe J, Feudtner C. Navigating decisional discord: The pediatrician's role when child and parents disagree. *Pediatrics.* 2017;139(6):e20170234.

32 I Just Want to Feel Normal!

Jami Gross-Toalson and
Jennifer Linebarger

You are seeing a 17-year-old male who underwent heart transplant 4 years ago after developing acute cardiomyopathy. He is readmitted with rejection, and his medication levels are subtherapeutic.

The transplant team shares that his initial mild adjustment difficulties after transplant resolved. As he has aged, his parents have transitioned responsibility of his medication regimen to him, and they now only occasionally monitor the medications.

On admission, he reported missed and late doses of anti-rejection medications. His parents were unaware that this had been an issue. With questioning, the patient identifies that he feels a lack of control over his health. He also acknowledges disbelief that rejection could happen to him. Finally, he reports that he had difficulty adapting his medication regimen to fit into his active social and academic life and chose to avoid taking medications at prescribed times in order to feel "normal" like his peers.

What do you do now?

ADHERENCE AND NONADHERENCE

Like so many things in medicine, the difference between compliance and adherence is subtle and emphasizes the importance of involving the patient in their care. Compliance is about how the patient *complies* with the prescriber's recommendations; the patient plays a passive role in the prescription. Adherence incorporates the patient into the decision-making and recommendations, and it requires the patient's agreement to the recommendations. Noncompliance is generally used to suggest a patient's intentional refusal; nonadherence incorporates a complex range of factors leading to a patient's ability to follow treatment recommendations.

The World Health Organization suggests there are five dimensions to adherence:

- Social and economic factors—such as literacy, costs, distance from health services, cultural barriers, and age/development
- Health care team and system-related factors—including patient–provider relationship and insurance
- Condition-related factors—including the level of disability and disease severity
- Therapy-related factors—such as the complexity, side effects, or changes in the regimen
- Patient-related factors—starting with the patient's knowledge and beliefs about their illness

Struggles within any of these dimensions can contribute to nonadherence. There are significant potential health complications resulting from nonadherence, such as hospital readmission, pain or worsening symptoms, higher health care costs, disease recurrence, and even death. Despite these risks, the rates of nonadherence to pediatric medical treatment are consistently found to be approximately 50–55%. Thus, identifying and intervening in cases of nonadherence are key to optimizing health in pediatric patients.

ASSESSMENT

Medication nonadherence should be considered whenever a patient's medical condition is not under control. Some recommend routine assessment in a blame-free environment to address concerns before the nonadherence impacts patient health. Patients are more likely to acknowledge difficulties with adherence when asked in a nonjudgmental manner. Perhaps start with a normative statement, such as "Being a teenager can make it difficult to do what you need to do to care for your health." Then move to questions such as the following:

· "Which dose of medicine is the hardest to take?"
· "Which part of your care is hardest to fit in to your daily life?"

Such questions can open the conversation to other barriers that impact how the patient is able to adhere to the treatment regimen.

Various measures of adherence have been utilized to allow for routine assessment of patient adherence. Often, a 24-hour recall of adherence is a strategy for providers to better understand typical strategies for patients to manage their health care in their normal environment. Pharmacy refill checks, missed appointments, and drug levels are additional strategies to better understand a patient's adherence. In addition, there are adherence-specific patient and family report measures that further delineate adherence concerns.

IDENTIFY BARRIERS

A key component of the assessment of a patient's adherence is identifying factors that serve as barriers to the patient following recommended medical treatments. The potential barriers to adherence for adolescents are numerous. There are both systematic and less formal strategies to assess barriers to adherence in the pediatric population. For example, Simons and Blount developed the Adolescent Medication Barriers Scale to allow for regular assessment of barriers to optimal treatment adherence. Using this measure, the authors suggest that barriers to pediatric adherence can be categorized into three primary types:

· Disease frustration/adolescent issues
· Ingestion issues
· Regimen adaptation/cognitive issues

Similar categories for adherence barriers have been delineated by other researchers and include emotional functioning, peer influences, self-efficacy, organization, financial issues, and social support. Whether these barriers are assessed systematically by validated measures or more informally by provider interviews, doing so allows the medical team to collaborate with adolescents and their families to alter how health care needs are met and minimize barriers to treatment adherence.

MOVING FORWARD TOWARD IMPROVED ADHERENCE

Once a blame-free assessment leads to barrier identification, work can begin on improving treatment adherence. Such work is a collaborative effort with the patient, parents, and treatment team. Interdisciplinary supports to address specific barriers can be put in place. For example, mental health treatment may be needed to minimize the impact of depression or anxiety symptoms on adherence, as well as to improve overall adjustment to the health condition. Working with the physicians and pharmacists can assist in decreasing the complexity of a regimen that is too complicated to be accurately followed. Enlisting parents in monitoring medications more closely, despite the desire for autonomy of adolescents, may minimize the impact of forgetfulness.

Some patients may demonstrate improved adherence simply by helping them identify what makes adherence difficult for them. This insight into what is not going well in regard to self-care of medical needs may serve to motivate the patient to improve upon their health care self-management. However, many others may require more intensive interventions based on a thorough assessment. Mental health screening is one important way to ensure that adolescents are receiving the supports necessary to live their lives as healthy as possible. Patients with depression or anxiety, both of which are prevalent in adolescents with chronic health conditions, may demonstrate avoidance of their health care needs or a lack of motivation to care for themselves. These comorbid mental health concerns will not be resolved simply by awareness but, rather, require a referral for intervention by appropriate mental health professions.

Adolescents with chronic health conditions may also struggle with the balance between living their lives as a normal adolescent and the health care needs that make them feel different from peers. At a time in life in which peers have a major influence, adolescents may choose peer acceptance over health without fully recognizing the long-term consequences of this choice. By assisting these patients in identifying their goals both for their health and for their life in general, the team and family may be better able to help the adolescent move forward in a way that allows him or her to make healthy choices while also assimilating with peers. When possible, connecting adolescents with other peers who have similar health conditions may help normalize their experience, as well as allow them to discuss adherence concerns and learn from others how they have managed similar issues. In addition, problem-solving training to assist in learning to balance health care needs with other priorities can be beneficial to adolescents.

For adolescents who struggle with organization and managing a complex regimen, they may benefit from technology to improve adherence. Given the prevalent use of smartphones and tablets, adherence-focused apps are often useful in helping adolescents better maintain adherence. These apps are beneficial due to their proximity and availability to the patient throughout the day. In addition, many of them allow for autonomy in managing health care needs while also providing a way for parents or other caregivers to monitor or participate in the health care treatment. For patients who do not rely on technology, reminders can be developed using a daily planner, sticky notes, and other behavioral strategies and cueing.

Including parents in the health care regimen, especially for older adolescents, can be difficult for many reasons. Parents may believe that their adolescent should be old enough to manage their health care independently. There may be parent–child discord related to poor adherence. Finally, adolescents may want to be autonomous but lack the necessary skills to do so. In each of these cases, it is important for the medical team to reassure parents of their important role in supporting their adolescent but also helping them understand the importance of facilitating developmentally appropriate autonomy. Several strategies are available to include parents without having a negative impact on the parent–child relationship. Reducing the parents' inclination to punish adolescents for poor adherence may improve communication and allow adolescents to feel more comfortable acknowledging when they need help. It can also be beneficial to help parents learn to be a "safety net" for their adolescents, monitoring adherence without being the primary reminder or person responsible. This "assisted independence" allows the adolescent to learn how to meet their own health care needs with support and help when they need it.

For the teenage patient in the case example, assessment identified that his barriers were related to "disease frustration/adolescent issues." Appropriate interventions to address these struggles include involving parents in medication adherence support in a developmentally appropriate manner, modifying the treatment regimen in a way that minimizes its impact on his social life and allows him some "control," and counseling to help address emotions related to his health history and its impact on his life.

KEY POINTS TO REMEMBER

- Nonadherence incorporates a complex range of factors leading to a patient's ability to follow treatment recommendations.
- Patients are more likely to acknowledge difficulties with adherence when asked in a nonjudgmental way.
- Common barriers to treatment adherence include disease frustration, adolescent development, medication regimen issues, and cognitive or mental health concerns.
- A collaborative team approach can create a safety net to support the patient's treatment adherence.

Further Reading

Greenly RN, Stephens M, Doughty A, Raboin T, Kugathasan S. Barriers to adherence among adolescents with inflammatory bowel disease. *Inflamm Bowel Dis*. 2010;16(1):36–41.

Hanghoj S, Boisen KA. Self-reported barriers to medication adherence among chronically ill adolescents. *J Adolescent Health*. 2013;54(2):121–138.

Logan D, Zelikovsky N, Labay L, Spergel J. The Illness Management Survey: Identifying adolescents' perceptions of barriers to adherence. *J Pediatr Psychol*. 2003;28(6):383–392.

Rapoff MA. *Adherence to Pediatric Medical Regimens*. 2nd ed. New York, NY: Springer; 2010.

Simons LE, Blount RL. Identifying barriers to medication adherence in adolescent transplant recipients. *J Pediatr Psychol*. 2007;32(7):831–844.

World Health Organization. *Adherence to Long-Term Therapies: Evidence for Action*. Geneva, Switzerland: World Health Organization; 2003. Retrieved from https://www.who.int/chp/knowledge/publications/adherence_full_report.pdf

33 I Need a Refill

Elissa G. Miller

You are called by an oncologist in your hospital about a patient she is seeing in clinic. She tells you that her patient is undergoing treatment for a solid tumor that was fully resected a few months ago. He has persistent pain but had been stable on non-opioid medications plus low-dose opioid as needed. However, recently his opioid requirement is increasing, and today he is asking for a refill of his oxycodone 2 weeks early. The oncologist is worried he may be misusing his opioids and wants to know what you recommend.

What do you do now?

SUBSTANCE MISUSE AND ABUSE

Patients may request an early refill of controlled substances for a number of reasons. However, the two most dangerous reasons—drug abuse and drug diversion—are what we worry about when a patient such as the one in the case example presents to clinic.

Drug misuse is use of a substance in a manner other than its intended or prescribed purpose. An example of substance misuse is taking more of a medication than was prescribed—either taking it more frequently than prescribed or taking a larger dose than prescribed. Patients undergoing cancer treatment or other painful treatment may be at risk for this type of substance misuse, especially if they are underreporting their symptoms to their care team or if the care team is undertreating reported symptoms. The patient in our scenario may be misusing his opioid medication and putting himself at risk without realizing it. More than 20% of patients who misuse opioids report getting the prescription from a doctor, and another 50% of patients who misuse painkillers report getting them from a friend or relative. Obtaining medication from a friend or relative is known as drug diversion. Drug diversion is the transfer of any prescribed controlled substance from the individual for whom it was prescribed to another individual. So our patient could be misusing his opioids, but he could also be diverting them—giving them away or selling them.

Drug misuse and diversion may seem harmless, especially if they are done rarely and the drug is obtained with permission of the owner. And many teens believe that prescription drugs are safer than street drugs because they are prescribed by a doctor. However, frequent misuse can lead to drug abuse.

Drug dependence refers to physical dependence on a substance. Dependence is characterized by the symptoms of tolerance and withdrawal, and it is common among patients for whom controlled substances are prescribed. However, drug dependence and misuse may lead to drug abuse or substance use disorder (SUD). SUD is marked by a pattern of repeated substance use that often interferes with health, work, or social relationships. Death rates from opioid overdose have been increasing in the United States in recent years (Figure 33.1). Although multifactorial, this is due in part to opioid overprescribing by clinicians: 80% of heroin users report first misusing prescription opioids. For this reason, monitoring for misuse

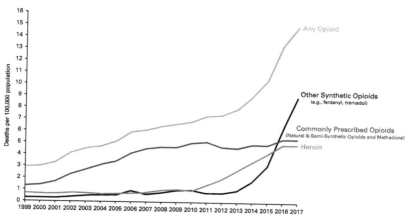

FIGURE 33.1 Death rates involving opioids.

Source: CDC/NCHS, National Vital Statistics System, Mortality. CDC WONDER, Atlanta, GA: US Department of Health and Human Services, CDC; 2018. https://wonder.cdc.gov.

should be standard practice for all physicians who prescribe controlled substances.

UNIVERSAL PRECAUTIONS FOR OPIOID PRESCRIBING

Universal precautions for opioid prescribing involve a standard set of practices that are recommended for use by all practitioners with all patients when prescribing opioids for chronic pain management. Having a standardized approach helps keep patients safe; minimizes the risk of patients feeling judged by their provider; and, by treating everyone the same, takes provider judgments about who is "likely to misuse" or who is "trustworthy"—judgments that are based on conscious and unconscious biases and therefore inherently flawed—out of the encounter. Universal precautions also help provide objective data, which becomes helpful if concerns for misuse, abuse, or diversion arise.

The components of universal precautions for opioid prescribing are shown in Table 33.1. The most difficult part of universal precautions to adapt to pediatric care are the assessment tools, which are not validated for pediatric use. These assessment tools also may be difficult to apply for patients who are nonverbal or for children whose parents are reporting all

TABLE 33.1 **Components of Universal Precautions for Opioid Prescribing**

Item	Reasons for Use	Commonly Used Tools	Frequency of Use
Patient functional assessment	Helps set realistic treatment goals that are based on function rather than the total elimination of pain	PEG—Pain, Enjoyment of Life, General Activity Questionnaire FRQ—Functional Recovery Questionnaire	With every visit
Psychological assessment	Assesses for depression, a condition that can worsen pain, and if left untreated, may put a patient at risk for opioid misuse	PHQ-9—Patient Health Questionnaire–9 GAD-7—General Anxiety Disorder Questionnaire–7 AUDIT—Alcohol Use Disorders Identification Test DUDIT—Drug Use Disorders Identification Test	At treatment initiation and again if concerns arise
Risk assessment	Provides an evidence-based method of determining a patient's risk of substance misuse and abuse	ORT—Opioid Risk Tool SOAPP® and SOAPP®-R—Screener and Opioid Assessment for Patients with Pain and Revised SISAP—Screening Instrument for Substance Abuse Potential CRAFFT tool	At treatment initiation

TABLE 33.1 **Continued**

Item	Reasons for Use	Commonly Used Tools	Frequency of Use
Risk stratification	Helps providers know their patients' risk of opioid misuse and helps establish frequency of follow-up		Annually
Urine drug screen	Monitors to ensure patients are using the medications prescribed and to ensure they are not misusing or abuse other substances		Minimum: At treatment initiation and then every 6 months Also use if concerns arise, such as patient appears intoxicated in clinic or pill counts are not correct
Controlled substance agreement	Sets clearly defined expectations from the outset of treatment Describes up front the conditions under which the prescriber may stop prescribing opioids		Annually

(*continued*)

TABLE 33.1 **Continued**

Item	Reasons for Use	Commonly Used Tools	Frequency of Use
Prescription drug monitoring program check	Allows providers to view all controlled substance prescriptions to ensure patients are not receiving medications from multiple sources		Minimum: Every 6 months Ideal: With every controlled substance prescription
Pill or patch count	Strategy for monitoring appropriate opioid use by assessing quantity of pills or patches remaining compared to expected quanity		Every visit following initiation of therapy
Substance misuse assessment	Assesses risk of substance misuse for patients receiving chronic opioid therapy	COMM—Current Opioid Misuse Measure PDQP-p— Prescription Drug Use Questionnaire– patent ABC—Addiction Behavior Checklist	Every visit following initiation of therapy
Naloxone co-prescription	Reversal agent in the event of accidental over-dose		Consider at treatment initiation

medical information. However, these children and families must still be assessed because they are at risk for drug diversion by their caregivers. The Opioid Risk Tool (ORT) is validated down to age 16 years, and the Car, Relax, Alone, Forget, Friends, Trouble (CRAFFT) tool is validated for use in children aged 12–21 years. For younger children and for those who are nonverbal, an adaptation from Cincinnati Children's Hospital Medical Center may be applicable:

- Does anyone in the child's home or the patient have a history of drug abuse (yes or no)?
- Does anyone in the child's home or the patient have a history of mental health problems (yes or no)?

The remainder of the components of standard opioid prescribing precautions can be applied across the age and developmental spectrum.

PAIN CONTRACTS/CONTROLLED SUBSTANCE AGREEMENTS

A unique component of universal precautions for opioid prescribing is the pain contract or controlled substance agreement (CSA). This is a document signed by the patient or legal guardian for those younger than age 18 years (often the parent) and the provider. CSAs may vary across practices; however, they typically contain the same key content sections. These are an agreement that the patient

- receives their opioid prescription from a single prescriber or prescriber group;
- fills their opioid prescription at a single pharmacy;
- does not miss or cancel follow-up clinic visits with less than 24-hours notice;
- brings all pill bottles to every visit for pill counts;
- agrees to undergo routine urine drug screen (UDS);
- agrees not to misuse or divert their medications;
- agrees not to use or misuse other prescription or nonprescription substances; and
- understands that violation of the contract may result in no further opioid prescriptions.

These agreements may be time-consuming to discuss; however, when used up front at initiation of opioid therapy, they help educate regarding the risks associated with use and misuse of prescription opioids and stress the importance of adherence to the treatment plan.

DISCONTINUING OPIOID THERAPY

The decision to discontinue opioid therapy may be due to one of a few reasons: Opioid treatment is not improving patient function (i.e., opioids are not helping), opioid treatment is no longer clinically indicated due to resolution of pain, or a patient is unable to adhere to a safe treatment plan and the risk of further opioid prescribing outweighs the benefits. The third possibility—a patient is at greater risk with continued opioid therapy than without—is often a difficult situation for everyone involved. Providers worry that patients will be angry with them or that they may harm a patient by discontinuing opioid therapy. Patients may become angry and/or fearful that their pain will worsen in the absence of opioid therapy. It is important for providers to remember that we may abandon opioid therapy but should not abandon our patients. Continuing to see a patient even after the discontinuation of opioid therapy when the discontinuation is due to concerns for opioid misuse should be standard for any physician who is seeing a patient for chronic pain management. Continuing with adjuvant pain management—pharmacologic and nonpharmacologic therapies—is important in helping manage chronic pain. The patient, however, may choose not to continue seeing the provider.

If discontinuation of opioid therapy is due to substance misuse or concerns for abuse, such as a patient who presents to clinic intoxicated, the patient should be informed of the reason, assessed for substance use disorder, and referred for treatment as clinically indicated. In the case of our patient, his oncologist is concerned about opioid misuse. You see the patient, and after completing a history and physical exam, you realize that this patient has pseudo-addiction. Pseudo-addiction resembles drug addiction in that patients use more medication than prescribed, run out of prescriptions early, and may be seen to be drug seeking. However, it is not caused by the psychological disorder of addiction. Rather, it is due to underprescribing of medications to treat pain. Patients with untreated pain will seek more medication in order to obtain pain relief. You increase your patient's total daily opioid, initiate long-acting opioid therapy, and complete the entire universal precautions for opioid prescribing package, including risk assessment, prescription drug monitoring program (PDMP) check, UDS, CSA, and psychological health screening. You find nothing concerning on UDS and PDMP check, and your patient screens low risk for opioid abuse on the ORT and negative for depression on the Patient Health Questionnaire–9 (PHQ-9). A Pain, Enjoyment of Life, General Activity Questionnaire (PEG) scale shows this patient's pain is severely impacting his daily functioning. You see him 4 weeks later for follow-up and to prescribe refills. He reports significantly improved functioning with his long-acting opioid. He is using zero or one as-needed doses of opioid daily and brought his pill bottles to the clinic visit as instructed. After initiating adjuvant pain management, including gabapentin, and cognitive–behavioral therapy with a pain psychologist, and physical therapy 3 days per week, your patient improves significantly, and you are able to wean his long-acting opioid after just a few weeks of use while upholding his CSA.

KEY POINTS TO REMEMBER

- Universal precautions for opioid prescribing should be used for all patients who are starting opioid therapy that is expected to be chronic/continued use.
- Pediatric patients are at risk for substance misuse and abuse, and these patients and those who are most vulnerable are at risk for drug diversion by their caregivers or family members.
- Discontinuing opioid therapy due to concerns for opioid misuse or abuse may be necessary.

Further Reading
CRAFFT. Retrieved June 29, 2019, from http://crafft.org
Ehrentraut JH, Kern KD, Long SA, An AQ, Faughnan LG, Anghelescu DL. Opioid misuse behaviors in adolescents and young adults in a hematology/oncology setting. *J Pediatr Psychol*. 2014;39(10):1149–1160.

Thienprayoon R, Porter K, Tate M, Ashby M, Meyer M. Risk stratification for opioid misuse in children, adolescents, and young adults: A quality improvement project. *Pediatrics*. 2017;139(1).

Volk K. *Teen Prescription Drug Misuse and Abuse*. Rockville, MD: Substance Abuse and Mental Health Services Administration; 2016.

Webster LR. The prescription drug abuse epidemic and emerging prescribing guidelines. In Benzon HT, Raja SN, Liu SS, Fishman SM, Cohen SP, eds. *Essentials of Pain Medicine*. Philadelphia, PA: Elsevier; 2018:389–394.

34 They're Taking Away Her Health Insurance!

Cory Ellen Nourie

A 17-year-old female is admitted with recurrent aspiration pneumonitis. Her past medical history is significant for cerebral palsy with spastic quadriplegia, a 120-degree neuromuscular scoliosis curve, delayed gastric emptying with associated gastroesophageal reflux disease, and jejunostomy tube-dependent feeding. Her mother is hesitant to proceed with the anterior and posterior spinal fusion that the orthopedist has recommended for several years, citing the risks while also acknowledging that her daughter's quality of life will continue to deteriorate as her curve continues to worsen. She lives at home with a single parent, who wants her daughter to continue to live at home as long as possible but references ongoing caregiver stress and lack of home health supports. Her mother mentions her daughter is losing her Medicaid coverage with her upcoming birthday and wants to know how to navigate care without it.

What do you do now?

TRANSITION TO ADULT CARE

The prospect of transitioning to services in adult health care services can be confusing and frightening for families as they leave the pediatric care they have come to know and trust. Disruption in services and supports during this transition period is a common experience, and advanced planning is crucial. With proper guidance, it is possible for some patients to retain services and government benefits, such as Medicaid, long term. The conversations around transition preparation and planning should begin with pediatric patients in their mid-teen years. Due to the difficulty with prognostication for children with complex chronic conditions, it is advisable to conduct transition planning to adult services for these patients to avoid a crisis point at adulthood.

One of the most essential aspects of transition planning is to ensure the family has conducted special needs estate planning. Although older adults may be familiar with estate planning, it is common for most to be unaware of special needs estate planning, especially in states where this resource is scarce. Special needs estate planning revolves around the young adult's access to, and eligibility for, government benefits. Although the pediatric palliative care patient may have a limited life span compared to their typical peer, eligibility for services can be dramatically impacted or altogether eliminated by a nonexistent special needs estate plan. The first key part of special needs estate planning is to understand government benefits and eligibility for them. For teenage/young adults with chronic conditions or special health care needs, their medical condition may make it difficult or impossible to obtain meaningful employment. Although their employability may be challenged, their expenses and need for income do not stop. Young adults who are not able to work more than 20 hours a week in gainful employment may be eligible to receive Supplemental Security Income (SSI) from Social Security. Once patients turn 18 years old, they are considered adults and can apply for adult SSI. In order to be eligible for SSI, the person with a disability cannot have more than $2,000 in assets in his name. This includes all bank accounts, stocks, bonds, and so on. If the person has more than $2,000 in his name, he will automatically be determined to be ineligible for SSI. As part of the special needs estate planning process, a family member may choose to establish a special needs trust or an Achieving a

Better Life Experience (ABLE) account on behalf of the person with a disability. These are the only two ways a person who is otherwise eligible for SSI may save more than $2,000 in his name. It is essential that families work with a certified special needs estate planner and attorney to fully understand the options. Parents will often designate the special needs trust of their child with a disability as the beneficiary of life insurance policies, retirement accounts, or real estate. With those designations in place, if the parent (or other person who has designated the trust as the beneficiary) dies before the child, the money would go into the special needs trust, allowing the young adult to continue to access government benefits such as SSI. An ABLE account is the second way a person may save more than $2,000 in his name, but an ABLE account has annual maximum contribution limits as well as lifetime limits before it impacts one's SSI payment amount. Most states use the same definition criteria for SSI as they do for Medicaid eligibility, so most young adults with SSI automatically receive their state's Medicaid as insurance. This is one of the key reasons special needs estate planning is essential; so the pediatric patient does not lose access to health insurance as an adult. Interestingly, for the pediatric palliative care patient, a special needs estate plan may also include information about resource distribution from the young adult's estate when she dies. These documents should be reviewed regularly and updated as appropriate.

Regarding the patient in the case example, she needs to apply for SSI when she turns age 18 years, which once approved will continue to allow her to have Medicaid as her insurance. Medicaid in adult health care has different parameters for accessing home nursing, and in her case, she needs to opt into the long-term care Medicaid to continue to have home nursing supports.

Another important consideration for pediatric palliative care patients as they make the move to adult services and supports hinges on their legal status and the age of majority. In most states, the age of majority is 18 years; however, you may want to double check in your state. Once patients turn age 18 years in the United States, the Health Information Portability and Accountability Act (HIPAA) takes effect, which gives all decision-making power to the individual. HIPAA also states that providers cannot share medical information with anyone, without the permission of the individual patient. HIPAA does not bar family members from sharing information with providers; it limits providers' ability to share information without consent of the adult patient. HIPAA is not supposed to be a barrier in continuity of care, so if a patient has invited another person to an appointment or procedure with them, it is implied that support person may have access to information from the provider in that situation, unless the patient expresses otherwise.

To prepare your patients, and their families, for reaching the age of majority, there are several considerations to know about. First, determine if your state has a health surrogacy law. This law automatically designates next-of-kin decision-makers for everyone older than age 18 years who are determined to not have capacity to make medical decisions, if no other decision-making document has been completed. For states with a health surrogacy law, families often feel less pressure to sign legal documents on the 18th birthday because the law appoints first a spouse, second an adult child, and third a parent as the decision-maker. In almost all these cases, this means the parent will be the decision-maker if their now adult child is not able to make or communicate healthcare decisions. The surrogacy law is a passive law, meaning it goes into effect if necessary. There are two other considerations concerning legal status, both of which require the patient and/or family members to proactively initiate a legal document. The two options are health care power of attorney and legal guardianship. Health care power of attorney allows any person older than age 18 years, who is capable of consenting to it, to appoint health care agents, who by their appointment are authorized to speak with the patient's health care providers on the patient's behalf, access the patient's records as necessary, and make medical decisions for the patient. Health care power of attorney can be made effective immediately or if/when the patient is determined to lack capacity. A health care power of attorney is a living document, meaning it can be edited and voided if necessary. Most teenage patients choose their parents, grandparents, or perhaps older siblings as their health care agents, but as they grow older they may decide to void the previous version and complete a new health care power of attorney appointing a spouse or close friend as the first decision-maker, and so on. It is important to note that even patients with intellectual disabilities may be capable of authorizing a health care power of attorney, using whatever form of communication they have to execute the document. Although the document has the word "attorney" in the title, developing a health care power of attorney document does not require an attorney to be involved. Every state has a health care power of attorney available for free online, usually as part of an advance directive packet. To be valid, the document must be notarized or witnessed by two people who are not part of their health care team. Once validated, patients should give copies to all of the health systems from which they receive care, as well as to their insurance companies. Having a health care power of attorney on file eliminates barriers to care, especially for young adults who are still navigating this newfound level of responsibility and still need the assistance of parents/caregivers. For patients older than the age of majority who do not have the ability to execute a health care power of attorney, obtaining legal guardianship requires a court proceeding in which the adult patient is determined to be legally incompetent to make decisions for him- or herself and a legal guardian is appointed to make all of their decisions. Legal guardianship is the most restrictive option because it is nearly impossible to reverse and is a permanent determination of incompetence. Once adult guardianship is in place, the guardian should consider who will assume the guardianship responsibilities if the guardian dies. If there is not someone willing or able to assume the guardianship, the legally determined incompetent person would become a ward of the state. Guardianship should be the last resort choice, after all other options have been considered. Legal guardianship also costs a significant amount of money, ranging from $750 to $14,000. In many instances, if a person has a profound intellectual disability, and the state has a health surrogacy law, then there is no need for guardianship because the health surrogacy law gives decision-making rights to the parents. Regarding our patient, she has intellectual disabilities and uses an augmentative communication device to communicate. When she turns age 18 years, she can execute a health care power of attorney to allow her mother to continue to be part of her health care team, giving her access to communicating with her providers and authorizing her mother to make decisions for her if she cannot. If she lacks capacity when she turns age 18 years, the state's surrogacy law would apply, and her mother would be her automatic surrogate decision-maker. Your state's protection and advocacy agency or disability law program are good resources to offer for further discussions.

For patients moving into adult services, it is important for them to register with their state agency for intellectual developmental disabilities or the office of aging and adults with physical disabilities if they may need ongoing supports for living. Each agency has specific criteria for eligibility. If a young adult or family intend on the person living in a residential program, it is imperative they register with the agency because the wait list for residential services can be up to 10 years. Parents are aging at the same rate as their now-adult child with disabilities and chronic conditions, and caregiving burdens become more obvious. If the intention is for the young adult to live at home indefinitely with family members, accessing funding for home health and personal care is through these state agencies and/or Medicaid. In addition, being registered with their state agency will open up access to case managers/care coordinators and potential job programs, volunteer opportunities, and other ways for the person to be part of their adult community.

Planning for transfer of care from pediatric to adult healthcare for a palliative care patient takes time and careful planning. In an ideal situation, pediatric providers will identify and communicate with their adult counterparts to conduct a detailed discussion of the patient's plan of care. The primary care provider in the adult health care system is a key person in this transition period. The care model in pediatrics tends to be specialty based, whereas in the adult system, the primary care provider directs the care, with specialists providing consultation. Identifying a primary care provider with expertise and comfort in pediatric-onset conditions is most useful. Having ongoing dialog with the new providers, while the patient is still managed by the pediatric team, will reduce gaps in care. The transition from pediatric to adult palliative care teams is essential to plan and coordinate as well. Services may vary between the two systems, including members of the team and their responsibilities. For instance, pediatric palliative care may have child life specialists as team members, whereas adult palliative care may not. It is important to have multiple, ongoing conversations with both the patient and the family, as well as the new adult team, to create as smooth a process and eventual transfer as possible. Co-managing or overlapping services and supports makes for a more gradual transition, in which the new providers become accustomed to the patient's needs and the previous team transfers knowledge to the new provider. Programs supporting young adults in the transition process, for both medical and nonmedical care, are becoming more prevalent throughout the United States. In some cases, pediatric palliative care patients may be granted an exception to allow a dying patient to finish their life with the pediatric team.

KEY POINTS TO REMEMBER

- Families who have members with disabilities/chronic medical issues should meet with special needs estate planners to create estate plans and wills that protect the patient's access to long-term government benefits, including SSI and Medicaid.
- When they reach the age of majority, patients should designate their health care agent through a health care power of attorney if possible. If they do not have capacity to complete this form, families should consider their state's health surrogacy law or legal guardianship if necessary.
- Patients should be connected with their state's disability agency to access supports and services in the adult system, including home health care. There are often wait lists for these services, so registering in their teen years is recommended.
- Transferring to adult providers should be planned in advance, with deliberate identification of adult providers. Direct conversations between the pediatric team and the adult team should occur for successful information sharing.

Further Reading

Got Transition/Center for Health Care Transition Improvement. Retrieved May 24, 2019, from https://www.gottransition.org

Nemours Children's Health System. Becoming an adult: Legal and financial planning. Retrieved May 24, 2019, from https://www.youtu.be/CpvlyfiRjRM

Nemours Children's Health System. Becoming an adult: Taking more responsibility for my care. Retrieved May 24, 2019, from https://www.youtu.be/cjXurYrFMZM

Nemours Children's Health System. Becoming an adult: What can I do after high school? Retrieved May 24, 2019, from http://www.youtu.be/gdFb4NsifAM

Nemours Children's Health System. Becoming an adult: Deciding where to live. Retrieved May 24, 2019, from http://youtu.be/8bBp3VX71Hs

US Department of Health and Human Services, Administration for Community Living. State protection & advocacy systems. Retrieved from https://acl.gov/programs/aging-and-disability-networks/state-protection-advocacy-systems

Special Considerations

35   The Unexpected Question

Amelia Hayes

You are caring for a 20-year-old female with acute
myeloid leukemia. She underwent a bone marrow
transplant; however, her post-transplant course has
been more complicated than expected with multiple
setbacks, including now viral sepsis. Your patient
progresses to multisystem organ failure and is now
intubated and sedated in the intensive care unit. The
medical team believes that she has no reasonable
chance of recovery. She is single, and her mother is
her surrogate decision-maker.

"She would not have wanted to live like this," her
mother says. "I do not want to put her through any
more, and I think I should let her go." After making the
most difficult decision of her life, she turns to you and
says, "I do not know how to tell my other children.
Can you do it?"

What do you do now?

TALKING TO CHILDREN ABOUT DEATH

There is no doubt that talking to children about death is stressful for anyone. A common response from medical providers is to call the social worker or call the child life specialist and let them handle this conversation. However, when other resources are not available to you, what do you do? As a medical provider, you need to be comfortable having these conversations because they will inevitably happen throughout your career. In addition, if you have a supportive and trusting relationship with the family and they are most comfortable with you, you may be the most appropriate person to have this conversation.

So where do you start? First, gather the facts:

- How old are the siblings? Are they developmentally where you would expect?
- What comforts them? What helps them when they are upset? Any triggers you should avoid?
- What do they know already? How does their mother expect them to react?
- What language have the parents or other caregivers used with them?
- Do they have a faith or belief system that will affect their thinking about withdrawing technology or what happens after death?
- What will her death look like—calm and peaceful or more distressing?
- Will they want to see her before she dies, and if so, is her mother okay with that?
- Does her mother or another family member want to be present for this conversation?

In this case, you have never met her siblings, but you find out from her mother that they are all brothers aged 13, 8, and 6 years. The brothers are close knit and developmentally appropriate. They often play together, enjoy video games, and their mother thinks they will be a good support to each other. They know that their sister has cancer, but the family has not discussed death or even the possibility that their sister could die. Your patient's mother is feeling anxious about the conversation, is not sure how they are going to react, and decides she does not want to be present during the conversation. Because she is not going to be present, you know you must have a good idea of the family belief system prior to the conversation because there will not be anyone there to correct any mistakes you may make. You find out that they are a religious family, and her mother tells you about their beliefs as they relate to death. Her mother is okay with the brothers coming into the room after your conversation to see their sister, and you find out they have been to visit many times already and have seen her in her current state, so her intubation and the multiple medication infusions will not be a shock to them. Next, you check in with the medical team, and they believe her death will be peaceful and they will be able to keep her comfortable with little or no additional distress for the family to witness.

At this point, you have a basic understanding of the family structure and beliefs, but you also need an understanding of the typical response and understanding of death for children in her brothers' age groups. This is important to know because children are unpredictable and may have many questions for you or they may have none. It is essential to address any common fears or misconceptions, whether or not they ask, because more than likely children are thinking about them even if they cannot verbalize them. Children have active imaginations, and often their imaginations are much worse than reality. If we do not address common fears, and they are too uncomfortable or unwilling to ask, we have left them with nothing but their imaginations to rely on. Table 35.1 lists grief responses in children by age.

Now that you are fully prepared to talk with the siblings, you need to find a space to do so. A quiet corner in the unit playroom normally works well because there will be something for the siblings to engage in immediately after the conversation or when/if they cannot process any more and need a break. A quiet and private conference room will work as well, and you can grab a few distraction items to bring along with you just in case they are needed. Finally, you know that this will not be an easy conversation and do not know how long it will take, so ensure you have someone to cover your other work for you so you are not interrupted.

TABLE 35.1 **Grief Responses in Children by Age Range**

Age Range	Responses
Infants	Have no concept of death, but will sense changes in the emotions of adult caregivers.
2–4 years	Believe the world revolves around them. Death is viewed as abandonment. Tend to ask repetitive questions about deceased (e.g., "Did you know my daddy died?" "When will he be home?")
4–7 years	Fantasy and magical thinking. Death viewed as reversible. May believe they caused the death with their thoughts or actions.
7–11 years	Beginning to think logically and understand that death is final. May view death as punishment. Fear pain and bodily harm. Will often hide feelings.
11–18 years	Abstract thinking—can take a more adult approach. Trying to come to terms with what death means for them.

Now you have the brothers in the playroom. You are by yourself with them, and they are looking at you. What do you say? You know this conversation is going to change their lives, so you take it slow and simple:

I have some news I would like to share with you about your sister. I know you have been to visit her many times and know that she is really sick, what else do you know about how she is doing?

Giving the brothers a space to tell you what they already know allows you to assess their understanding, find out what misconceptions you will have to clarify, and takes the burden off of you to have to explain things they already understand (this can also be a useful tool when talking directly with sick children). Her oldest brother states that he knows she has cancer but that her transplant is not going well. He knows that the tube in her mouth is helping her breath and that she is on many medications. Her other two brothers do not have anything to say. You state,

You are absolutely correct. All of the doctors here have been working really hard to help your sister through this transplant, and you are right it is not going well. We have been giving her all of our best medications and they are not working. Her body is really sick and now we are worried that the medicines we have been giving her are hurting her and not helping her. After talking it over with your mother, we have decided together we are going to stop those medications today that are not helping her and just give her medicines that will make her comfortable and make sure she is not in any pain. After we do this, we think she will die this afternoon.

It is important to emphasize that you are still caring for their sister and not giving up on her. You are still going to make sure she is comfortable and not in pain. It is also important to make sure you do not place blame on the caregivers. You do not want to leave the siblings with the feeling that their mother decided to give up, does not care anymore, or is responsible for the death of their sister. During this incredibly difficult time in their lives, you need to preserve those caregiver relationships.

At this point in the conversation, the siblings have gone quiet. The 6-year-old brother does not seem to be paying attention and is coloring quietly. The 8-year-old brother is tearful and not making eye contact with you, and the 13-year-old brother is stoic. Because you have a mix of ages, you want to clarify that they understood what you meant. So you ask, "Do you know what it means to die?" The 8-year-old brother, who now has his arm around the 6-year-old brother, states that his sister will go to heaven. The 13-year-old brother states that she will not be with them any-more. You tell them,

That is right, she will not be with you anymore. Her spirit will go to heaven but that also means that her body will stop working. Her heart and other organs will not work anymore. She will not breathe anymore and will not be able to feel any pain.

You use the terms "spirit" and "heaven" because their mother had indicated that this was their belief, but it is also important to indicate concretely what happens to the body. Although it may seem harsh in the moment or diffi-cult to talk about body mechanics not working anymore, you know that her 6- and 8-year-old brothers could still fall into magical thinking and may not yet grasp the finality of death. In addition, although it may be difficult for you to say, it is worse for her brothers to think she is potentially breathing and/or feeling things while buried after death. You are also intentional in avoiding the use of common euphemisms for death, such as "passed away," "went to sleep," "gone," or "lost." These euphemisms are confusing for children and often end up creating more distress. When you ask if they have additional questions, they report they have none. Before you leave the brothers, you know it is important to address potential fears even if they are not expressing any. You state,

> I know that this is really hard. You guys are great brothers and I just want you to know that there is nothing you did that caused this. You did not do anything wrong and I am sorry that this is happening. I wish that our medications had helped, but her death is not related to anything that any of you did, said, or thought.

The siblings are not saying much, and you are sensing they need a break. You know that children grieve at their own pace, and they would probably like to get back to something normal such as play. You remember that their mother mentioned they liked video games, and you get them set up playing a game together. You then return to update their mother on the conversation.

You tell the mother that the siblings took the news as well as you would expect and that they were tearful and quiet. You tell her that you explained to them what it meant to die, and you share some of the words you used so she can use the same if they ask additional questions later. Table 35.2 gives detailed examples of how children at various ages, like her children, grieve and how she may be able to help each of her children as they process the news they heard today. Although you believe they understood everything in the moment, you know that her younger siblings especially will need repetition to fully understand. As a way to improve processing and coping with this news, you suggest getting them involved with art and music activities because these can help children process emotions indirectly. You also let her know that it is okay if the siblings see her cry or get upset, and she does not have to hold back emotion in front of them. This lets them know that emotions are okay and gives them permission to express theirs as well. Finally, you suggest that she give them some time to play and then go check on them and allow them to go see their sister if they wish.

TABLE 35.2 **Understanding Grieving Children - By Age Group**

Age	Concept of Death	Grief Response	Developmental Stage/Task	Signs of Distress	Possible Interventions
2-4	Egocentric; believes world centers around them; narcissistic; no cognitive understanding; pre-conceptual; unable to grasp concepts	Seen as abandonment; seen as reversible, not permanent; common statements, "Did you know my daddy died?" When will he be home?"	Intensive response but brief; very present oriented; most aware of altered patterns of care; repeated questions	Regression; changes in eating and sleeping patterns; bedwetting; general irritability and confusion	Short and honest interactions; frequent repetition; comforting; reassurance; nurturing; consistent routine.
4-7	Gaining sense of autonomy; exploring world outside of self; gaining language; fantasy thinking and wishing; initiative phase seeing self as initiator; concerns of guilt	Death still seen as reversible; great personification of death; feeling of responsibility because of wishes and thoughts; common statements, "It's my fault. I was mad at her and wished she'd die."	Verbalization; great concern with process; How? Why?; repetitive questioning; may act as though nothing has happened; general distress and confusion	Regression; nightmares; sleeping and eating disturbances; violent play; attempts to take on role of person who died	Symbolic play using drawings and stories; allow and encourage expression of energy and feelings through physical outlets; talk about it

(continued)

TABLE 35.2 **Continued**

Age	Concept of Death	Grief Response	Developmental Stage/Task	Signs of Distress	Possible Interventions
7-11	Concrete thinking; self-confidence develops; beginning of socialization; development of cognitive ability; beginning of logical thinking	Death as punishment; fear of bodily harm and mutilation; this is a difficult transition period, still wanting to see death as reversible but beginning to see it as final	Specific questioning; desire for complete detail; concerned with how others are responding; What is the right way? How should they be responding?; starting to have ability to mourn and understand mourning	Regression; problems in school, withdrawal from friends; acting out; sleeping and eating disturbances; overwhelming concern with body; suicidal thoughts (desire to join one who died); role confusion	Answer questions; encourage expression of range of feelings; encourage and allow control; be available but allow time alone; symbolic play; allow for physical outlets; Talk about it
11-18	Formal operational problem solving; abstract thinking; integration of one's own personality	"ADULT" approach; ability to abstract; beginning to truly conceptualize death; work at making sense of teachings	Depression; denial; repression; more often willing to talk to people outside of family; traditional mourning	Depression; anger; anger toward parents; non-compliance; rejection of former teaching; role confusion; acting out	Encourage verbalization; do not take control; encourage self-motivation; listen; be available; do not attempt to take grief away

*Courtesy of the Dougy Center for Grieving Children

Now re-imagine the scenario. This was an ideal situation in which you had the time to gather facts from the mother and prepare for the conversation. What if your patient was awake and asked you if she was going to die? What do you do now?

Often, the most intense questions from patients come when you least expect them. Thinking ahead of time how you would respond and having some sentences prepared can help you not feel overwhelmed when it eventually happens to you. All patients, but pediatric patients especially, are incredibly perceptive. They will sense the change in anxiety level in the room. They will notice when more conversations are happening outside of their room and not in their presence. They will notice when their parents look like they have been crying but say that they are fine. They will also notice when they seem to be getting away with more than they used to or are receiving more gifts than normal. So when a patient asks you if they are going to die, they have probably been thinking about it for awhile. They are searching for someone to be honest with them, and as uncomfortable as it may be, we owe them an honest response. The following are suggestions for potential ways to respond when a patient asks, "Am I going to die?" (choose the most honest):

- "What made you think about that? I have no reason to believe right now that that will happen. I will let you know if that changes."
- "What made you think about that? I am worried that you could die from your disease, but we are doing everything we can to try and prevent that. Would you like to talk more about that?"
- "What made you think about that? I am worried that you will die from your disease. We will do everything we can to make sure you are as comfortable as possible. Would you like to talk more about that?"
- When you need to gather more information: "That's a great question. What other questions have you been thinking about? Let's write them all down and I'll come back and answer them all for you in a little while."

Talking with sick children and their siblings about death is important and must be done well and at a developmental level that is appropriate for the children involved.

- Go slow and be honest. Start with short and simple explanations, and allow the child to guide the conversation. Answer the questions asked without elaborating unless prompted by the child. Allow the child to lead the conversation, ask open-ended questions, and reflect back what they say to assess their understanding.
- Be concrete and aware of developmental issues. Be aware of normal developmental fears and be sure to address them. Use concrete language even if it feels uncomfortable for you, and avoid euphemisms.
- Displays of emotion by adults are okay. Despite this, parents are often uncomfortable crying in front of their children. However, when parents share their feelings and emotions, it gives their child permission to do so as well.
- Give space for expression. Not all children are going to cry and be sad like we might expect them to be; some will return to play quickly and act like nothing happened. Allow space for children to grieve at their own pace. Art, music, and books are often excellent modalities for children to address their emotions indirectly.

Further Reading

Schneider L. 10 things grieving children want you to know. Eluna Network. Retrieved October 2018 from https://elunanetwork.org/resources/10-things-greiving-children-want-you-to-know

Sisk BA, Bluebond-Lagner M, Wiener L, Mack J, Wolfe J. Prognostic disclosures to children: A historical perspective. *Pediatrics*. 2016;138:e20161278.

The Dougy Center. Developmental grief responses. Retrieved October 2018 from https://www.dougy.org/grief-resources/developmental-grief-responses

The Dougy Center. Tips for supporting grieving children. Retrieved October 2018 from https://www.dougy.org/grief-resources/tip-sheets/tips-for-supporting-grieving-children/1660

The Sharing Place. A child's concept of death. Retrieved October 2018 from https://www.thesharingplace.org/docs/Concepts_of_Death.pdf

The Sharing Place. Understanding grieving children—by age group. Retrieved October 2018 from https://www.thesharingplace.org/docs/Grief_by_Age_Groups.pdf

36 A Winding Path

Meghan L. Marsac

You are caring for a 17-year-old male in treatment for
rhabdomyosarcoma. He has a very close-knit family,
including his father, mother, sister, and brother. His
father was identified by the family as the decision-
maker for medical care; his father rarely attended
appointments. When he did attend, he frequently
presented with anger and stated that "my son will
be fine." Your patient's mother was identified as
responsible for overall care of their children, including
medical care; she generally focused on caring for her
son while avoiding talking about his cancer and her
own feelings. Younger siblings were rarely mentioned
and were not integrated into medical care. Your
patient's most recent biopsy suggested a terminal
relapse of rhabdomyosarcoma; at this news, his
mother (alone in the waiting room) burst into tears.
His father hung up the phone on the medical provider
who contacted him with biopsy results. His mother
does not know what to tell her son or his siblings.

What do you do now?

ANTICIPATORY GREIF AND BEREAVEMENT

Quite often, each individual within a family unit will experience anticipatory grief and bereavement differently. In your patient's case, we observe family members with some similar and some different anticipatory grief reactions related to his diagnosis and prognosis. Both parents exhibit some symptoms of avoidance in how they manage his medical care, converse with medical professionals, and communicate within the family. The avoidance allows the parents to retain a layer of self-protection to process their son's disease and eventual death more slowly over time, at their own pace. Whereas your patient's mother outwardly displays more sadness about the loss of her son, his father expresses his emotions surrounding the expected loss as anger. Although we do not know how siblings are experiencing his disease process and anticipated death, based on common sibling reactions, they are likely incurring mixed emotions that may include feelings of loss of the prior relationship that they had with their brother, worries and/or sadness for their brother, sadness or anger at missing time with their mother, and possibly jealousy of the attention their brother is now receiving. Because your patient's siblings have been provided with very little information about their brother's disease and prognosis, they have been left to try to figure it out on their own; this often leads to misunderstanding and additional fears. Siblings may also be tasked with taking on more household responsibilities and trying to "be perfect" so that they do not add to their parents' stress. In this family, each family member is expressing feelings associated with current and anticipated loss; these feelings often ebb and flow as the disease progresses and continue following the patient's death.

Anticipatory grief is defined as loss experienced prior to death; this can include the loss of hopes or dreams over time. For example, in your patient's family, the parents had to grieve the loss of seeing him graduate high school and starting a family of his own; they also had to face feelings about changes to their parenting role. Rather than parenting their child into an independent life, they instead are forced to parent him through his death. Siblings had to grieve the loss of the sibling relationship that they once had and possibly the one person who understood what it was like to grow up in their family.

Bereavement includes the grief experienced following death; bereavement lasts a lifetime and fluctuates in its expression over time. The grief experienced within bereavement can vary substantially for individuals, even within the same family. For example, based on their initial reactions to your patient's disease, although both of your patient's parents may experience continued avoidance or denial as part of their grief process, it is likely that his mother will express her grief through sadness while his father may express his grief through anger, at least in the early aftermath of his death. Bereavement reactions can be triggered at any time, sometimes even by positive life events; for example, parents may experience reactions during holidays or when another child starts school or gets married. Sometimes the anniversary of a diagnosis or death can bring renewed feelings of grief.

In considering both anticipatory grief and bereavement, differential diagnoses to consider include persistent complex bereavement disorder, post-traumatic stress disorder (PTSD), major depressive disorder (MDD), and generalized anxiety disorder (GAD). Many emotional health symptoms can present as individuals experience grief/bereavement, and these additional mental health disorders should be considered on a case-by-case basis. Symptoms should be interpreted in the context of their severity and also in the context of what would be expected given cultural norms. Monitoring symptoms over time to determine if their severity persists can be helpful in deciding whether a diagnosis of a mental health disorder is warranted.

In persistent complex bereavement disorder, individuals may experience intense grief for a prolonged period of time that interferes with daily functioning. In this disorder, individuals continue to yearn for the loved one who has died, with the intensity of this yearning continuing over time rather than decreasing as would be expected. For your patient's family, intense grief would be normative in the weeks to months following his death; however, we would expect his siblings to be able to return to school, his father to work, and his mother to managing their household. If grief persists or worsens over time, complex bereavement may be considered. Similar to complex bereavement, PTSD related to the death of a loved one includes a preoccupation with the loved one but focuses on traumatic aspects of the loss rather than the loss of the person (e.g., for your patient's mother, the news of the relapsed cancer could serve as a traumatic event). In PTSD, individuals may experience intrusive thoughts about their loved one's death or a traumatic aspect of their loved one's disease or death. They also may avoid reminders of the death, such as certain medical providers or the hospital.

In examining depression, those experiencing grief will often experience a depressed mood in waves, triggered by memories of the loved one; this differs from MDD, in which an individual will experience a persistent depressed mood and inability to enjoy activities. In addition, those experiencing a depressed mood in response to grief are often able to maintain their sense of self and worth, whereas those experiencing MDD may experience feelings of worthlessness. For example, if your patient's mother's sadness is primarily related to his death, and she is still able to enjoy time with his siblings or have times in which the depressed mood lifts, she is more likely experiencing sadness in the context of bereavement rather than MDD. However, if her sadness begins to consume her life, she may be experiencing MDD along with bereavement. For GAD, anxiety generalizes beyond events related to the child's medical care and death. It is worth noting that those experiencing normative bereavement may also have co-morbid emotional health challenges that may create additional complexity in recovering from or accepting their loss.

Medical teams have the opportunity to help family members grieve in an adaptive manner. Ideally, medical teams are staffed with multidisciplinary team members to maximize the child's physical health and the child's and family's emotional and spiritual well-being. Medical teams can provide anticipatory guidance to families on normative grief processes and early bereavement. These conversations can start well before end-of-life conversations because many families experience anticipatory grief throughout the treatment of a serious disease. The medical team can also support the family through early bereavement by checking in and remaining a part of the family's supportive community.

For every family, medical teams should work to optimize communication between medical team members and family members. Medical teams may want to consider how each family best receives information. For example, does the family trust a certain team member? Does the family need information in writing to help them review and process it over time? Do certain family members need to be included in every communication? Communication with families about their goals of care and how to maximize quality of life and minimize suffering can also help families as they prepare for the child's death. Difficult information (e.g., change in prognosis, progression toward end of life, and a change in the treatment plan) should be handled with even more care, having primary providers deliver this information or be present when this information is shared, whenever possible.

Medical teams also have the opportunity to support within-family communication. Many parents find it challenging to share difficult information with their children (including the patient and siblings). Medical teams may want to identify team members who can work with this specific challenge for families. Often, psychosocial team members such as child life specialists, social workers, and psychologists are well trained to support within-family communication, including providing education for siblings. In educating siblings, teaching them about their brother's or sister's medical condition prior to end of life can be helpful. Part of this education can also include normalizing grief reactions to prepare them for what to expect and to help them accept their own potentially complicated feelings. It may also be beneficial to guide siblings in identifying supportive people (in addition to their parents) and in coaching them on how to ask for support when they need it.

Medical teams may also want to create handouts to review with family members that focus on normalizing emotional challenges and offering local or online resources. Families have expressed that having primary medical team members present during death can be very helpful; thus, trying to arrange for at least one primary medical team member to be available during or soon after death may be beneficial for the family. Families often become close with their medical team as part of their supportive community; having a bereavement program or procedures in place to follow up with the family in the weeks to months following death can serve as an additional support to the family.

In addition to having strategies in place to support all families, treating providers can pay attention to factors that place family members at risk for longer term or more intense grief (Figure 36.1) and can consider integrating a screening tool into standard care. For example, although not developed specifically for palliative care/grief/bereavement, the Psychosocial Assessment Tool is a screener for parents that has been validated across

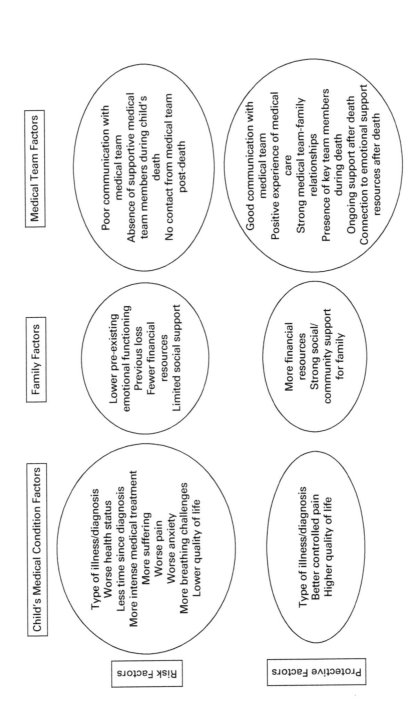

FIGURE 36.1 Factors affecting anticipatory grief and bereavement in family members.

numerous pediatric illness populations for its utility in identifying families with higher risk for challenges in psychosocial domains. If medical teams recognize more severe reactions (e.g., diagnosable mental health disorders or significant functional impairment), teams may want to encourage family members to seek an evaluation by a mental health counselor and/ or psychiatrist. In particular, if daily functioning (e.g., inability to go to school, work, parent, or otherwise achieve life goals) is impaired, additional services are warranted. Other factors that may place families at risk include intense medical treatment, substantially painful end-of-life path, challenging relationships with medical team members, and fewer financial resources.

KEY POINTS TO REMEMBER

- Anticipatory grief includes loss experiences prior to death, such as the loss of hopes and dreams for a child as well as the expected loss of life.
- Bereavement lasts a lifetime and fluctuates in its expression over time.
- The experience of grief is unique to the individual. Family members may grieve on different timelines and in different ways.
- Siblings are sometimes overlooked. Medical teams can help facilitate siblings' grief process by including them in discussions or providing parents with education on how to talk with siblings. Ideally, siblings learn about their brother's or sister's diagnosis prior to end of life.

Further Reading

American Psychiatric Association. *Diagnostic and Statistical Manual of Mental Disorders*. 5th ed. Arlington, VA: American Psychiatric Publishing; 2013.
Contro NA, Kreicbergs U, Reichard WJ, Sourkes BM. Anticipatory grief and bereavement. In: Wolfe J, Hinds PS, Sourkes BM, eds. *Textbook of Interdisciplinary Pediatric Palliative Care*. Philadelphia, PA: Elsevier; 2011:41–53.
Gao M, Slaven M. Best practices in children's bereavement: A qualitative analysis of needs and services. *J Pain Manage*. 2017;10(1):119–126.

Gerhardt CA, Baughcum AE, Fortney C, Lichtenthal WG. Palliative care, end of life, and bereavement. In: Roberts MC, Steele RG, eds. *Handbook of Pediatric Psychology*. 5th ed. New York, NY: Guilford; 2017:191–200.

Kazak AE, Schneider S, Didonato S, Pai AL. Family psychosocial risk screening guided by the Pediatric Psychosocial Preventative Health Model (PPPHM) using the Psychosocial Assessment Tool (PAT). *Acta Oncol.* 2015;54(5):574–580.

Marsac ML, Kindler C, Weiss D, Ragsdale L. Let's talk about it: Supporting family communication during end-of-life care of pediatric patients. *J Palliat Med.* 2018;21(6):862–878.

Richardson RA, Ferguson PA, Maxymiv S. Applying a positive youth development perspective to observation of bereavement camps for children and adolescents. *J Soc Work End Life Palliat Care.* 2017;13(2–3):173–192.

37 Why Is She So Distressed?

Daniel Waechter Webb and
Megan J. Thorvilson

You are caring for a 15-year-old star soccer player who was diagnosed with Ewing sarcoma of the right femur 2 years ago. She underwent chemotherapy and limb-sparing surgery and achieved remission. Just before the start of her soccer season, her positron emission tomography scan revealed concern for recurrence. She was admitted to expedite the evaluation. Her biopsy results are still pending, but since admission, her pain scores have escalated, despite reasonable doses of opioids. She is difficult to engage and always has the lights out and shades drawn when you enter the room. When she does engage, she reports nausea and requests lorazepam, which helped with nausea during her initial chemotherapy treatments. Her parents pull you aside in the hallway, expressing concern regarding her worsening symptoms, exclaiming, "You have to do something. She's just not herself. She won't accept any visitors. She's even avoiding social media."

What do you do now?

SPIRITUAL CARE OF CHILDREN AND TEENS

In medical contexts, children and families often face questions related to their humanity and life meaning. Spirituality serves as a key organizing principle in the midst of this vulnerability, connecting them to a wider sense of meaning-making, relationships with others, and relationships with the sacred/transcendent.

The realm of spirituality encompasses a range of human capacities and emotions, including a sense of wonder, a spirit of curiosity, and the weight of uncertainty. Spirituality permeates every dimension of children's lives, manifesting in play, curiosity, stories, and daydreaming. Yet, children often keep their spirituality private, and it may have an unpredictable relationship with the faith environment of their family. It escapes the standard faith categories of adults, requiring space for that which adults often do not understand or cannot imagine.

SPIRITUAL DISTRESS

Spiritual distress can be described as a disruption of one's ability to experience and integrate meaning in life. For medical providers who are attending and treating physical symptoms, it can be easy to overlook the spiritual dimensions of suffering. Spiritual distress can be difficult to identify because the well-being of the human spirit is often articulated through physical, psychological, and social means.

The physical challenges that serious illness imposes upon children create unique spiritual challenges. Pain can overwhelm the body, mind, and spirit. Disfigurement and loss of bodily functions and abilities are major transformations that cause confusion, anxiety, or despair. Children's image and experience of their bodies are an integral part of their sense of self, so in addition to the physical dimension of suffering, there is often a layer of spiritual distress rooted in the meaning children attach to what is happening. Spiritual distress can be expressed through physical symptoms, such as difficulty sleeping, nightmares, and crying uncontrollably. Whenever a child is unable to articulate spiritual pain, they may instead complain of somatic symptoms. No matter the source of spiritual distress, it is difficult for children to devote attention to their spiritual needs without sufficient pain and symptom management.

Spiritual distress is often expressed psychologically. Emotions are significant in the spiritual landscape for children, with fear and anxiety being particularly common and overwhelming. However, any emotion, whether positive or negative, can be a source of spiritual distress. Anger, bitterness, or guilt can be difficult to navigate, but positive emotions can be distressing if they are confusing or experienced in isolation from others. A child may not feel free to express happiness, relief, or celebration. The emotional state of a child can be a helpful indicator of spiritual well-being. If a child appears overwhelmed or unresponsive emotionally, it is worth considering spiritual distress as a source of suffering.

Social challenges can be particularly painful for seriously ill children, particularly isolation from family, friends, and community. Isolation can lead to feelings such as rejection, worthlessness, or loss that are deeply spiritual in nature. As children face the end of life, they may worry about being forgotten, grieve the loss of a future, or become anxious about the loved ones they will leave behind. Social indicators of spiritual distress include withdrawing from family members, friends, or other sources of support; displaying less interest in play and creative activities; and using more silence, resistance, or manipulation in relationships.

Relationships are of primary importance to children, so relational strains between parents/caregivers or between the child and a parent/caregiver can be some of the most challenging sources of spiritual distress for children and families. Holistic family-centered care recognizes the spiritual needs of children as well as their parents, caregivers, and siblings. One of the unique challenges of pediatric spiritual care is its relational nature. Children and parents each have their own spiritual needs, but these needs are interwoven in complex ways. Children may not express certain spiritual needs out of concern for their parents, and the same is true of parents concerned about their children.

ROLE OF SPIRITUALITY IN MEDICINE

Engagement with the spiritual realm in medicine is typically delegated to the chaplain, but that assumes too clean of a separation between medicine/health and spirituality. In reality, medicine and spirituality are far more intertwined. The majority of parents whose child died following a critical illness identified their spirituality as an important factor in their coping both in the midst of the illness and after the death of their child. Many parents used their spirituality to guide them in end-of-life decision-making, to make meaning of loss, and to sustain them emotionally. For parents, their primary spiritual concern was maintaining a connection with their child, especially during the dying process and after their child died. Parents would prefer to be open about their spiritual beliefs and practices with clinicians, but they rarely share this aspect of their experience, fearing a detraction from their child's medical care or perhaps judgment from the culture of science and medicine.

However, this fear may be unfounded because the majority of pediatricians recognize the importance of spirituality, acknowledging a positive role in healing, strengthening the therapeutic relationship, and providing support for patients/families. Despite that recognition, most pediatricians do not discuss spirituality with patients. This disparity likely stems from the lack of formal training around spirituality in medical education, the lack of a standardized tool to evaluate spirituality, and a personal discomfort with spirituality.

To help address this disparity, clinicians first can explore their own spirituality. Without a sense of comfort with one's spirituality, fear of the potential pain and anguish that may be expressed often prevents clinicians from addressing the altered spiritual needs of patients. Clinicians can then consider the spiritual needs of parents and pediatric patients separately. For parents, in the midst of a critical illness, spiritual needs include connection with the child, truth in communication, compassion, prayer/ritual/sacred text, connection with others, and bereavement support. They feel support from medical professionals through prayer, access to spiritual leaders, and a shared sense that the parent–child relationship endures despite death.

When considering the spiritual needs of children, clinicians must take great care not to conflate a parent's spiritual beliefs with those of the child. An understanding of the unique spiritual developmental needs of children can help preserve the rich distinction between children and their family unit.

SPIRITUAL NEEDS AND HUMAN DEVELOPMENT

The spiritual needs of children change and evolve as children grow and develop. While acknowledging that every child's development is unique, it is helpful to have an awareness of the general contours of spiritual development for each age group (Table 37.1). Keeping children's developmental

TABLE 37.1   Spiritual Needs in the Context of Child Development

Stage	Characteristics	Interventions
Infant	Nurturing environment supports basic trust in the world. Need for attachment. Engage the world by touch, sound, and taste. Sense impressions of the world cultivate sense that child is loved.	Encourage medically appropriate touch between caregiver and child. Use consistent care providers to promote trust. Hold, rock, and sing to baby.
Toddler	Need for play and use of motor skills. Control of body and movement provides sense of autonomy. Tactile exploration of the world. Repetitive behaviors build sense of achievement. Anxieties about strangers or separation from caregivers. May regress from previously acquired emotional and physical skills to cope (e.g., potty training or use of words).	Familiar toys, blankets, and comfort objects provide sense of security. Use games, toys, and art supplies in communication. Allow child to demonstrate what they do well. Normalize regressions that parents observe in child as part of child's coping.
Preschool	Developing language skills. Need consistency in schedule and rules when possible. Spirituality learned through stories and images. Child projects previous experiences onto new people, situations. Vivid imaginations are both fun and fearful. Fuzzy distinctions between reality and fantasy. Anticipatory fear. May believe illness is punishment. Child begins to participate more in prayers and religious rituals.	Encourage caregivers to read to child. Encourage caregivers to be consistent. Use stories in communication. Encourage children to tell their own stories. Look for emotions that may be expressed nonverbally or through dramatic play. Reassure child that illness is not a punishment. Encourage family to maintain religious rituals.

(continued)

TABLE 37.1 **Continued**

Stage	Characteristics	Interventions
School age	Takes pride in new responsibilities. Concrete thinkers. Emphasis on fairness, justice, reciprocity, and right and wrong. Building social networks at school. Aware of nonverbal cues and may understand more than adults realize. Open communication helps correct child's erroneous assumptions. Metaphors and symbols often taken literally. Deities are anthropomorphic (have human characteristics). Unanswered prayers can be particularly painful.	Consider that illness may create sense of failure or inadequacy. Look for feelings of isolation or anxiety about being different. Help child connect with peer group. Encourage emotional expression and open communication. Ask child what they understands. Use stories of superheroes or good vs. evil to connect with child's imagination.
Adolescence	Developing personal identity and independence. Need to be a part of decisions regarding their care. Questioning vs. conformity to religious authority. Attuned to expectations and judgments of others. Exposed to beliefs different from those of parents. Ability to think more abstractly. May look more to peers for support. Older adolescents hunger for romantic relationships. Struggle to find their own beliefs.	Teens may need space to differentiate from parents. Encourage communication with and connection to peers. Discuss their interests to build a connection. Allow child to articulate their hopes and dreams. Allow as many choices and as much control as possible.

context in mind is vital to connecting with them and attending to their needs. However, some experiences are essential to the well-being of children at any age—a sense of belonging, security, and belovedness. Yet even these core needs are communicated and felt in different ways as children grow. Caregivers and clinicians can use developmentally appropriate stories, music, and art to facilitate spiritual and emotional expression. Chronic life-threatening illness also limits a child's ability to experience their developmental context normally.

One way of viewing childhood spiritual development is to consider questions that might be particularly important for each age group:

- Infants depend on a sense of attachment to their caregivers. They learn whether they can trust the world around them from the way that caregivers respond to their needs. How can their environment and care promote a sense of safety and connection to caregivers?
- Toddlers thrive in tactile exploration of the world. In what ways can we provide opportunities for them to practice using motor skills or touch to explore the world and feel a sense of achievement or belonging?
- Preschool children are rapidly developing language skills as a way of understanding their own experiences and the world. What stories do preschool children like to hear and what are they communicating through the stories they tell? What stories might help them understand their experience of illness?
- Elementary school-age children typically understand the world in terms of fairness, right and wrong, and good and evil. Does their experience of illness cause confusion or spiritual pain within this black-and-white orientation? They may sense the acute unfairness of their situation and wonder why this is happening to them.
- Adolescents can think more abstractly and may articulate broader spiritual questions. Their relationship with their parents is evolving as well. How are they navigating any differences between their own needs and their parents' needs? How does their illness affect their friendships and social or romantic relationships? What experiences do they fear they will never have, and how do they cope with these fears and spiritual pains?

If we keep such questions in mind as we work to connect with children on their terms, we are more likely to notice spiritual distress and a greater range of emotional communication. The interventions offered in Table 37.1 are tips to encourage and equip parents as they seek to attend to their child's spiritual needs.

CONCRETE INTERVENTIONS

In conversations with parents and caregivers, medical providers can learn much about the caregivers' spiritual landscape, needs, and resources. Medical and spiritual languages often intersect in the ways that caregivers understand and explain health, disease, suffering, and healing. The priorities that parents articulate regarding the care of their children are often indicative of their spiritual values. It is also important to listen for the way that caregivers describe the place of physicians and medicine within their larger hopes and sense of faith.

One way to access the spiritual experiences and perspectives of caregivers is to ask questions that are not specifically medical in nature:

- How is your spirit today?
- What hurts your heart?
- What matters most to you right now?
- Is there anything that brings you a sense of peace in the middle of this?
- I can imagine that the decision you have to make is affected by your faith. Can you tell me more about that part of it?

When there are elements of spiritual distress that clinicians feel unprepared to address, there are resources available to explore the situation further. Chaplains can assess the spiritual needs of patients and families in greater detail and can be a resource when questions arise about spiritual concepts and phrases used by families. Chaplains can also bridge gaps in communication when spirituality is perceived as a barrier or when a family's spiritual beliefs do not align with the medical team's assessment of what is happening.

In addition to chaplains, child life specialists have a deep understanding of childhood development and regularly use therapeutic play and art techniques to help children express emotions. With this expertise, they have a unique and valuable angle on the spirit of the child. When available, child/pediatric psychologists are another valuable resource for supporting children and providing opportunities to cope with challenging emotions. For older children, adolescents, and parents, social media networks can be tremendous sources of spiritual support. Young people, who may otherwise feel isolated, often find social media a medium for self-expression, story-telling, or connection to others in similar circumstances.

The young woman in the case example demonstrated symptoms of spiritual distress. Any interdisciplinary team member has the potential to explore her distress. However, children and teens are most likely to reveal the sources of their distress to team members who have taken the time to build rapport and a relationship with them. Curiosity and compassion go a long way in building such bonds. Caring for any patient's spirit is a matter of trust. Working together as a team, clinicians can work to build networks of trust around patients and families. Through words, gestures, and presence, each clinician has the opportunity to care for the well-being of a person's body, mind, and spirit.

KEY POINTS TO REMEMBER

- As a key organizing principle in the midst of vulnerability, spirituality connects patients to a wider sense of meaning-making, relationships with others and relationships with the sacred/transcendent.
- Spiritual distress occurs when one's ability to experience and integrate meaning in life is disrupted, and can manifest in physical, psychological, and social ways.
- The spiritual needs of children change and evolve as children grow and develop.
- Chaplains, child life specialists, and psychologists can serve as supports to both patients and medical providers in the midst of spiritual discovery and distress.

Further Reading
Barton SJ, Selman L, Maslow G, Barfield R. Religion and spirituality in pediatrics. In: Balboni MJ, Peteet JR, eds. *Spirituality and Religion Within the Culture of*

Medicine: From Evidence to Practice. New York, NY: Oxford University Press; 2017:35–49.

Fosarelli P. Care of children. In: Cobb M, Puchalski CM, Rumbold B, eds. Oxford Textbook of Spirituality in Healthcare. New York, NY: Oxford University Press; 2012:243–249.

Foster TL, Bell CJ, Gilmer MJ. Symptom management of spiritual suffering in pediatric palliative care. J Hosp Palliat Nurs. 2012;14(2):109–115.

Meert KL, Thurston CS, Biller SH. The spiritual needs of parents at the time of their child's death in the pediatric intensive care unit and during bereavement: A qualitative study. Pediatr Crit Care Med. 2005;6(4):420–427.

Mueller CR. Spirituality in children: Understanding and developing interventions. Pediatr Nurs. 2010;36(4):197–208.

38 Maximizing the Time Left

Keith Pasichow

An 18-year-old female with progressive leukemia is referred to your service for discharge planning with home hospice. She has completed several rounds of chemotherapy with little response and has decided to focus on her comfort at this time. She reports nausea/vomiting, diffuse pain, lack of energy, and poor appetite related to nausea. Zofran has reduced her nausea, but she continues to have emesis one or two times per day. Her pain is diffuse, boney in nature, and constant with incident pain. It is worst in her lower back and hips and worsens with activity. She is mostly bed- or chairbound. She currently takes oxycodone 20 mg every 4 hours. She rates her constant pain as a 7/10 and incident pain as 10/10. The oxycodone reduces the pain to 5/10 and lasts for approximately 2 hours. Her goal is for her pain to be approximately a 2 or 3/10. She has been taking a number of other medications throughout treatments and would like to reduce these as much as possible.

What do you do now?

TRANSITION TO HOME HOSPICE

The transition from curative and palliative care to hospice can be a unique experience for pediatric patients and their families. The Medicare/Medicaid hospice benefit requires that a patient have a prognosis of 6 months or less, assuming the disease follows its common/natural course. However, because most patients will follow a unique path, many will live longer than 6 months and can remain on hospice as long as they continue to show evidence of a decline. As difficult as it is to prognosticate in adult medicine, it is even more challenging with pediatric patients, and so many of these patients may go on and off hospice several times as their disease progresses. There is no limit to the number of times a patient can sign off of hospice and then back on, provided they continue to meet the enrollment requirements. Most of the commercial insurance plans that pay for hospice use the Medicare criteria as well.

Patients transitioning from hospital-based palliative care to home hospice may go through a variety of emotions, including fear, depression, anger, and despair. They may be scared about changing a routine that has supported them for months, or even years, including doctor and hospital visits, disease-stabilizing or curative treatments, and important opportunities for socialization with peers in similar situations. Likewise, caregivers may be afraid of losing the supports and relationships they have developed during the time their child has been ill, including access to medical professionals and other families. During this time of transition, it is extremely important that the hospice team work closely with the patient and caregivers, as well as the hospital teams (disease specialists, palliative medicine teams, and psychosocial services), in order to smooth the transition and to engender trust in the new team on the part of the patient, caregivers, and medical teams.

It is very important to determine, as early as possible (preferably at the time of referral to hospice), who will be responsible for managing the patient's medications and other treatment modalities once the patient is at home. This responsibility may fall to the hospice medical director, the palliative care team from the hospital, the patient's specialist, or even the patient's primary care physician. Often, there is a collaborative approach because the palliative medicine team and hospice medical director will likely have expertise in managing difficult symptoms beyond that of other physicians or practitioners. In order to prevent miscommuniation or delay in medication management, this is one of the first issues that the hospice agency should clarify.

Regardless of who will be managing the patient's medications at home, an early assessment by the palliative care team and/or hospice team can be helpful to determine the caregiver resources. Will there be someone with the patient 24/7 or only a few hours each day? Can the patient manage their own medications, or will there need to be a caregiver present for any medication administration? Is the patient able to determine which as-needed medications are required and when/how to take them? Are there any concerns for medication misuse, abuse, or diversion in the household? Where will controlled substances be kept, and who will have access to them? Although a full discussion about tactics for minimizing the risk of diversion and abuse is beyond the scope of this chapter, this is an extremely important risk assessment to conduct at the time of hospice admission, if not sooner, so that a comprehensive plan can be put in place that protects patient access and provides patient and caregiver safety.

One major focus of a transition to hospice care is the optimization of comfort-directed therapies, and the discontinuation of any non-comfort-directed treatments, if this aligns with the patient's and the family's goals. Concurrent care allows for disease-directed therapies and hospice care simultaneously, in patients younger than age 21 years, who qualify for Medicaid or the Children's Health Insurance Program (CHIP). Transitioning a pediatric patient to hospice can be very different than that of the adult population. In the case example presented at the beginning of this chapter, the patient has requested that the hospice and palliative teams focus on her pain, nausea and vomiting, and appetite. Her current pain regimen is not working as well as she would like, nor is her antiemetic regimen. We may be tempted to make major changes in her palliative medications in order to get her symptoms under control as quickly as possible, but many patients have a particular attachment to the medications they have been using for long periods of time, and so it is important to determine the patient's and family's comfort level with making these changes. Pediatric patients in particular will often want to have a significant amount of control over these decisions, even in situations in which they may not be fully able to understand the impact of particular decisions. It is important to establish early in the relationship with these patients and caregivers who will be ultimately responsible for the decision-making, taking into account the local laws regarding age of majority. Keep in mind that a treatment regimen with which the patient is not in agreement will often not work as well as one that the patient has a sense of control over. Although this is true in any age group, adolescents and young adults in particular are trying to develop a sense of independence, hampered by their illness and the need for care provided by others. Giving them as much control as reasonable is an important part of their development and will help the medical team and the caregivers provide excellent comfort care during their time in hospice.

Once the assessment of the home, resources, and patient/caregiver preference for decision-making is complete, and the patient's and caregiver's comfort with medication changes is established, we can begin to create a treatment plan with the group. One of the most important parts of a hospice treatment plan is simplicity and ease of administration. Many patients will want to minimize the number of medications they need to take, as well as the frequency with which they take them. Often, a long-acting medication is preferred, especially with patients who may not have a caregiver 24/7 or when it may be challenging for the care team to give frequent breakthrough medications. Long-acting opioids, benzodiazepines, antipsychotics, and antiemetics are a powerful part of a home hospice team's toolbox and should be explored whenever appropriate. Furthermore, as a patient's disease progresses, they will often begin to have difficulty with oral medication administration such as pills or tablets. Part of a well-designed hospice plan of care includes a plan for transitioning to concentrated oral formulation medications that can be administered via sublingual, buccal, or even rectal routes when the need arises. Using medications that have an oral, liquid, and concentrated formulation available helps ease this transition. This makes the dosing and medication familiar to the caregiver and helps reduce the need for multiple medication changes as the patient nears the time of death. For refractory symptoms, or in cases in which the dose is too high to administer via the mucosa even with concentrated medications, hospice agencies typically have the ability to provide many comfort medications via subcutaneous infusion, including the use of patient-controlled analgesia machines to provide opioids safely and securely outside of the hospital.

Likewise, many medications that were used during the curative or stabilizing portion of the patient's treatment may be discontinued or weaned off in order to focus on the patient's comfort, avoid side effects, and polypharmacy. This process typically starts with medications that are least likely to have an impact on the patient's disease course, such as statins, and non-comfort-directed supplements, vitamins, and other medications that are only likely to have a long-term benefit for patients. A careful balance must be struck when deprescribing medications because some drugs may slow the progression of a patient's disease but may also cause significant side effects, such as steroids in patients with particular types of cancer or pulmonary disease. In these situations, collaboration with the patient's specialist or primary care physician is important and then a careful discussion with the patient and caregivers is critical to ensure that the patient understands the choices being made. Occasionally, patients or caregivers will choose to remain on a medication that may be causing some side effects if they determine that the beneficial effects of the medication outweigh the side effects. This is a very important time to include pediatric patients in the decision-making process as much as possible because they will likely have their own opinions about medications and side effects, including what is tolerable and what is not. It is important that the hospice team support these decisions but also be ready to make changes when the patient and caregivers are ready to do so or when the patient is no longer able to take the particular medication.

A unique aspect of home hospice is the emergency management plan. Although patients undergoing curative or stabilizing treatment will often be sent to the hospital when they have challenging breakthrough symptoms or emergencies such as fever, seizures, or refractory pain, the hospice philosophy is to keep the patient in their home or location of choice if possible. To this end, the plan of care for the patient cannot simply focus on existing symptoms but must also take into account the possibility of symptoms in the future. This requires a thorough knowledge of the common and not so common aspects of a patient's disease process, and close collaboration with the patient's disease specialist is often extremely helpful in this regard.

Hospice teams need to be prepared for symptoms the patient may experience as the disease continues to progress. Medications or a specific treatment modality should be easily available to the patient or caregiver to manage these anticipated symptoms. For example, in patients with central nervous system disease, seizures are a common part of disease progression; however, many of these patients will transition to home hospice without having had seizures and therefore without any experience managing them. Helping the caregivers and patients plan for the possibility of seizures is a key part of ensuring that these patients can remain at home throughout their time in hospice. Diazepam suppositories, lorazepam liquid, clonazepam dissolving wafers, and intranasal midazolam can be supplied in anticipation of a seizure. The key is to ensure that the patient has the medication in the home so that the team is not scrambling to find a 24-hour pharmacy at 2 AM when the patient is actively having an emergency. This philosophy is somewhat different from that of other fields of medicine in which 911 may be called or the patient may go to the emergency department. In hospice, although the patient is welcome to call 911 or go to the emergency department, the goal is to avoid this by managing all emergencies in the home, whenever possible.

Upon admission, hospice patients typically receive a comfort kit that contains frequently needed medications, such as liquid morphine concentrate, haloperidol, lorazepam, an antiemetic, and a cathartic for intermittent constipation. These kits can be supplemented with medications specific to the patient's disease process, such as the as-needed seizure medications mentioned previously, as well as medications such as risperidone for agitation or nausea and mirtazapine for insomnia.

While the medical portion of the hospice team is working on managing the patient's physical symptoms and developing a comprehensive emergency plan, the psychosocial members of the hospice team will be focusing on the psychosocial needs of the patient and caregivers. A unique aspect of hospice services is the provision of bereavement support for the caregivers after the patient has died. Currently, this benefit extends for 13 months from the date of death and can be extended further through referral to community resources for caregivers in need. This is particularly important in cases in which young children are part of the family unit and require developmentally appropriate support. The psychosocial aspect of the transition to home hospice is critical because many of the distressing symptoms patients have are made worse by anxiety, fear, and depression. The psychosocial members of the hospice team are an integral part in the development and updating of the hospice plan of care throughout the patient's time on hospice and are particularly important during periods of transition. Integration with members of the psychosocial teams in the hospital is critical to ensure the most comprehensive and effective treatment plan for the patient and caregivers.

–Pediatric patients who are able to, and wish to, should be allowed to have friends visit whenever possible. Part of the hospice plan of care may be the need for support for certain close friends of the patient, and the hospice team should collaborate closely with hospital psychosocial resources, as well as resources at school. Likewise, many pediatric, adolescent, and young adult patients are eligible for a wish through organizations such as Make-A-Wish and similar types of charities. If this has not taken place prior to the transition to hospice, the hospice team should make every effort to help make this referral if desired by the patient and caregivers. These final wishes take many different forms and can be therapeutic for the patient, caregivers, as well as close friends and relatives. They are also an important part of helping children, adolescents, and young adults transition through the disease and dying process.

As mentioned earlier in this chapter, concurrent care allows for pediatric patients on hospice to also receive disease-directed therapies, which is typically not allowed in adult hospice. This is unique to this pediatric population and creates many challenges for specialists and hospice providers. Whereas adult patients are required to forgo therapies with a curative intent upon enrolling in hospice (in most cases, although a few private insurance companies have similar concurrent care programs for adults. For these patients, it is extremely important for the palliative/hospice team to work closely with the treatment team because some palliative interventions may affect disease-directed treatment, and so decisions should be made jointly to avoid this when possible. Remember that for a patient to be eligible for hospice, they must have an estimated prognosis of 6 months or less, and this remains true whether a patient is receiving concurrent care or not. Thus, collaboration with pediatric palliative care specialists, where available, is particularly helpful in this population, in which patients may come off hospice for a period of time and still require palliative management.

- Close collaboration with treatment teams and existing palliative care teams is essential to creating a smooth transition to hospice.
- Deprescribing should be done in collaboration with the patient and caregivers and these changes should align with goals of care.
- Involve pediatric patients in discussions when they desire to participate and it is appropriate for their age and development. Involvement may help them be more at ease with the treatment plan.

Further Reading

Keim-Malpass J, Lindley L. End-of-life transitions and hospice utilization for adolescents. *J Hosp Palliat Nurs.* 2017;19(4):376–382.

Lockwood B, Humphrey L. Supporting children and families at a child's end of life. *Child Adolesc Psychiatric Clin North Am.* 2018;27:527–537.

Price J, McCloskey S, Brazil K. The role of hospice in the transition from hospital to home for technology-dependent children—A qualitative study. *J Clin Nurs.* 2018;27:396–406.

Index

Tables, figures and boxes are indicated by *t*, *f* and *b* following the page number
For the benefit of digital users, indexed terms that span two pages (e.g., 52–53) may, on occasion, appear on only one of those pages.